FOOD ALLERGIES
MADE SIMPLE

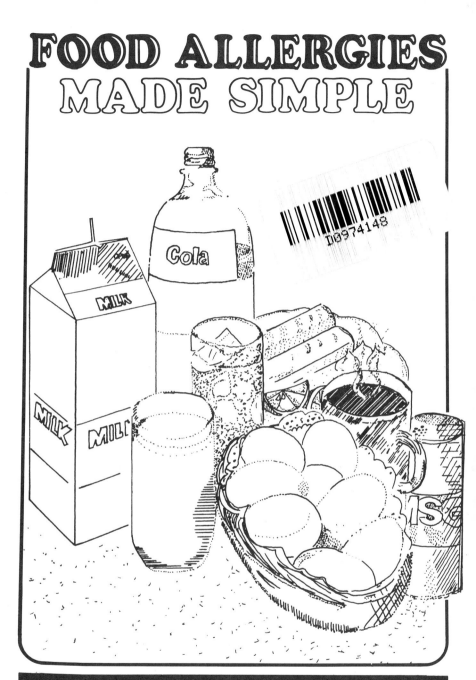

**Phylis Austin · Agatha Thrash, M.D.
Calvin Thrash, M.D.**

Food Allergies Made Simple

Phylis Austin
Agatha Thrash, M.D.
Calvin Thrash, M.D.

Family Health Publications
8777 E. Musgrove Hwy.
Sunfield, MI. 48890

Library of Congress Cataloging in Publication Data

Austin, Phylis
  Food allergies made simple.

  Bibliography: p.
  Includes Index.
  1. Food allergy. I. Thrash, Agatha M., 1931-
II. Thrash, Calvin L., 1928-   III. Title. [DNLM:
1. Food Hypersensitivity – popular works. WD 310 A937f]
RC596.A87 1985   616.97'5   85-3174
ISBN 1-878726-05-6

Table of Contents

CHAPTER ONE

What is an Allergy?

The word "allergy" comes from two Greek words: allos, which means "other" and ergon, which means "work." A simple definition of allergy is "reaction to a harmless substance." For many people this substance has no adverse effect, but in others, for reasons not yet fully understood, the body's defenses over-react to these substances, somewhat like calling the fire department to put out a burning match.

The function of the immune system is to protect us from disease. Each cell in our body has special markings which indicate that the cell is a part of us. Special white blood cells, called lymphocytes, constantly travel throughout the body looking for enemy invaders. When foreign cells or any kind of foreign substances are discovered the lymphocytes send chemical messages which summon macrophages (another type of white blood cell) to "eat up" the invaders.

For some reason, not yet understood, the immune system sometimes reacts to harmless invaders, resulting in an illness which we call an allergy.

An allergen (also called an antigen) is a substance which produces an allergic reaction. An antibody is a substance produced by the body in response to an allergen.

When a person with allergy is exposed to an antigen his body responds by producing antibodies. The antigens and antibodies combine to release chemical compounds in the body.

The body must produce sufficient antibodies before an allergic reaction will occur. For this reason a person generally does not react the first time the person is exposed to the substance.

Now we may make our definition of allergy more precise by saying that it is an abnormal reaction to a generally harmless substance, occurring in a predisposed individual, and caused by an antigen-antibody union. All of this process results in the release of histamine and other reaction substances, to be discussed later.

Bacteria which invade the body are made of various chemicals which form distinctive patterns and shapes on the cell surface. Antibodies are proteins made up of amino acids. When a germ enters the body, antibodies are produced that fit together with the bacterium (antigen). A "pat-

1

tern" is kept for those antibodies produced and should the antigens ever invade the body again the template is ready for the production of antibodies. This is what gives us immunity to some diseases once we have been exposed to them.

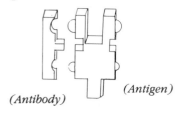

(Antibody)   (Antigen)

The Antibody fits the Antigen like a key fits a lock.

Antibodies are immunoglobulins of five different types: IgG, IgM, IgA, IgD, and IgE. Most of the immunoglobulins in the human blood are of the IgG type. Their main function is to protect the body from viruses and bacteria, and toxins. They appear after the macroglobulin (IgM). The IgA globulin is called "secretory" as it is seen primarily in bodily secretions – saliva, tears, gastrointestinal and respiratory mucus and breast milk. IgD is present only in small amounts, and its function is not yet clearly understood. Macroglobulin, the IgM globulin is the first seen after an infection or immunization. It serves as a natural antibody against toxins formed by intestinal bacteria. IgE globulin has only recently been discovered, and is found in very small quantities.

IgE is the globulin responsible for allergic reactions. These molecules are "Y" shaped, and the tail attaches to special sites on the surface of particular cells called mast cells. The arms of the "Y" may grasp antigen molecules; two adjoining "Y" arms may hold the same antigen, to form a bridge. The formation of the bridge stimulates the chemical packages inside the mast cells to empty their contents.

Histamine is one of the main chemicals released by the mast cells. Histamine and other chemicals released in response to allergy have a variety of effects on the human body. The blood capillaries widen and allow fluid to leak out into the body tissues. Smooth muscle under the influence of histamine may contract, stimulating the mucus-producing cells. An allergic reaction in the nose, such as occurs in hay fever, causes the nasal membranes to swell and become watery. Itching and tearing result from an allergic reaction in the eyes. Hives may result from an allergic reaction in the skin, cramps and diarrhea may result from an allergic reaction occurring in the stomach and intestine.

Interestingly, the same allergen may produce different symptoms in different people. In one person an allergy to milk may produce constipation, in another diarrhea, in a third, headache or bizarre thoughts, in a fourth cough or asthma. The organ affected is referred to as the "shock organ."

FAMILIAL TENDENCY

Allergies tend to run in families. If both parents have allergies a child has nearly a 75 percent chance of having a food allergy. If only one parent is allergic the child has a 50 percent chance. People who are allergic are often referred to as "atopic."

A child has a greater chance of developing allergies if he is exposed to cigarette smoke.

A food allergy may change expressions as the person ages. In a newborn, cow's milk may produce colic, in an infant cow's milk may produce eczema, at two to three years of age he may suffer asthma, as a teenager, acne and as an adult this same person may suffer migraine with the use of milk.

Sometimes food allergies appear in cycles, with periods of clearing alternating with periods of symptoms. As time passes the symptomatic periods become longer and closer together and may eventually become constant.

A person with a food allergy is likely to also have an allergy to other substances such as mold, chemicals, animal dander or dust. Food allergy is not an isolated disease and these substances must be taken into consideration when testing for food allergies.

ALLERGY VERSUS SENSITIVITY

Traditional allergists often object to the use of the term "food allergies" to describe many of the varied symptoms that can occur with this syndrome. They would prefer a rather rigid definition of an allergy, and would want to see predictable elevations of immune globulins in the blood. Others insist that the food-related symptoms cannot be so narrowly circumscribed. Perhaps one way to resolve this dilemma would be to use the term "food sensitivities" instead of allergies, as a sort of catch-all term. In this book, since we are speaking mainly to persons other than allergists, we have generally used "food allergies" as a general term to describe most of the symptom complexes related to foods, whether due to antigen-antibody reactions or to other, often poorly understood mechanisms. Most of the time the term food allergy and food sensitivity are used interchangeably.

CHAPTER TWO

Food Allergy – A Common Problem

FOOD INTOLERANCE IN 60% OF HUMAN ILLNESS

We have often heard it said that one man's food is another man's poison, and this certainly applies to food allergy. An article in Parade Magazine for August 1, 1982 states that food intolerances are involved in 60 percent of all human illness.

Food allergy may appear early in life or even be present at birth. (34) While other types of allergy may be "outgrown," food allergy often persists the entire lifetime. New food allergies are acquired along the way, and old ones may worsen. Avoidance is the only treatment for food allergy; hyposensitization has been shown to be ineffective.

Symptoms produced by food allergy range from only occasional minor discomfort to life-threatening anaphylaxis. They may begin on the day of birth, or at any time during the life. There may be only one symptom or a combination of symptoms, and symptoms of food allergy often resemble symptoms of other diseases.

A person may sometimes tolerate a food if he eats it only once every four to fourteen days. The frequency with which a food is eaten enters into its allergenicity; the more often it is eaten the more likely a person is to develop an allergy to it.

A CAUSE AND A TRIGGER

A food may produce symptoms on one occasion, but not on another. Some foods must be eaten in certain amounts to produce symptoms, and sometimes occur only in connection with other events. For example, some people react to melons only during the ragweed season. Some foods eaten raw produce symptoms, but eaten after cooking produce no symptoms. This is particularly true of apple, carrot, tomato, melon, and banana. (34) Cooking changes the structure of foods, sometimes making them less allergenic.

ADDICTION OR CRAVING?

People sometimes dislike the food they are allergic to, and refuse to eat it. Others crave the food. Craving occurs so frequently that some allergists actually replace the word "allergy" with "addiction." A person may develop a type of withdrawal symptoms if the food is discontinued, and insist that eating the food actually makes him feel better. As early as 400 B. C. Hippocrates observed that people were sometimes "injured" by changing their diet. He was referring to the "withdrawal" symptoms common to this type of addiction.

IMMEDIATE AND DELAYED SYMPTOMS

There are two types of food allergy. The first type is of immediate onset with symptoms appearing within seconds or minutes of eating the food. Anaphylaxis (shock), urticaria (hives), angioedema (swelling of skin), and asthma may be common symptoms with the immediate onset type. Egg, nuts, peanut, fish and shellfish are foods that often induce immediate onset of symptoms.

The other type of food allergy is the delayed reaction type. Symptoms may appear hours or even days after the food is eaten. Symptoms such as tiredness, irritability, paleness, leg aches, bedwetting, headaches, colic, poor concentration, diarrhea, bronchial asthma, rhinitis, indigestion, gas, headache, depression, hyperactivity, insomnia and dermatitis are usual in the delayed reaction type of allergy. Milk, chocolate, legumes, citrus, and food additives are commonly responsible for delayed onset symptoms. Because of the delay in onset of symptoms it is difficult to associate the use of the food with the allergic symptoms. (36)

Other factors may make delayed onset symptoms difficult to recognize: the response may vary from exposure to exposure; symptoms are often bizarre, and they may be due to additives or hidden ingredients rather than to specific foods. If a food is prepared without these additives no symptoms result, making diagnosis still more difficult. Wheat treated with pesticides may induce symptoms, untreated wheat may not. Milk sold in cornstarch coated containers may induce symptoms while bottled milk may not. Burgers fried in a teflon pan or broiled in a gas oven may produce symptoms but the same food prepared in an electric oven may not.

VARIABLE SYMPTOMS CONFUSE DIAGNOSIS

Symptoms may be intermittent even when the amount of food remains constant. Foods taken in small amounts may induce minimal symptoms, but if large amounts are taken, particularly after a period of not using the food, symptoms may be quite dramatic.

A patient may develop one symptom in response to several different foods, or different symptoms with different foods.

Because symptoms may be bizarre allergic people are often considered neurotic. These patients may be unable to cope with life problems because they are distracted by their allergic symptoms. They are sometimes encouraged to take vitamin and mineral supplements, or tranquilizers, which only perpetuate the problem.

MASKING

Sometimes a patient may take an allergenic food daily or even several times a day without being aware of any symptoms of allergy. He may even eat the food frequently because it makes him feel better. The symptoms may be delayed two or three days, so the patient rarely suspects it. If he stops the use of the food for four or five days, and then reintroduces it, there may be a marked reaction. The patient may begin to suspect that he is indeed allergic to this food so he decides to deliberately eat it again to see if the symptoms occur a second time. This time there may be no allergic reaction, so the patient concludes that he is not allergic to that food. What has actually happened is that the first set of symptoms have "masked" the second. If the food is eaten for the second time within 72 hours of the first consumption, the symptoms have not completely subsided, and hide the second series. If the food is not introduced into the diet for 72 hours, the initial symptoms will subside, allowing symptoms to reappear at the second ingestion.

When a person leaves off a food he is allergic to he may feel worse for the first couple of days. This is similar to symptoms of drug withdrawal. After two to three days the increased symptoms will subside and the person begins to feel better.

FACTORS PREDISPOSING TO FOOD ALLERGY

General good health measures such as sunlight, fresh air, exercise, rest, proper cleanliness, etc., may assist the body's immune system to cope with allergens.

Heredity plays a major role in food allergy. Age at the time of onset of the allergy may determine the severity of the symptoms; the younger the person is at the onset the more extensive is the allergic reaction. While there are no major differences in allergies between males and females, women may note worsening of symptoms immediately before and during the first day or so of their menstrual cycle. Alcohol and aspirin both increase the severity of allergic symptoms. Infections such as whooping cough, infectious mononucleosis, measles, influenza, peritonitis, and bronchopneumonia may precipitate food allergies, or worsen those symptoms already present. High humidity, fatigue, cold weather, and chilling may lower tolerance to allergens. Some people have improvement during the summer months with worsening of symptoms during winter.

How quickly a food is eaten enters into the intensity of the symptoms. A food eaten over a period of five minutes may produce more severe symptoms than if it were eaten over a 45 minute period. This may have to do partially with how well a food is chewed. If properly chewed, 98 percent of protein is absorbed as small peptides and amino acids. (44) If the food is consumed in a liquid form symptoms may be of shorter duration than those of the same food eaten in a solid form.

SYMPTOMS OF FOOD ALLERGY

Food allergy may produce a broad spectrum of signs and symptoms. No disease now known to medical science has the potential for producing a greater variety of symptoms.

Chronic fatigue and weakness are often due to food allergy. They may remain even after the obvious allergic attack subsides, and may become the patient's chief complaint. The fatigue due to food allergy may be worse in the morning and immediately after arising, and frequently appears in the mid – or late-afternoon. No amount of rest relieves the fatigue. Children who are difficult to awaken in the morning may rise in a good mood after the allergens are removed from their diets.

Aching, tightness, and pulling of the muscles of the shoulders, neck, and back, which may or may not be associated with headache may persist for days or weeks. Backache, arm, and leg aches may occur after ingestion of allergenic foods.

Enlargement of the lymph glands of the neck and cervical area associated with fatigue, and enlarged tonsils may be relieved with allergy management.

Mental symptoms such as tenseness, nervousness, irritability, quarrelsomeness, stubborness, restlessness, inattentiveness, jitteriness, stuttering, incoherent speech, lethargy, dullness, aphasia (inability to speak), and a feeling of having been drugged are common in allergic individuals. Depression, discouragement, and melancholia may also be noted.

Authorities feel that 95% of all migraines are due to multiple food sensitivities. Non-migraine headaches may also be caused by allergens.

Eczema, angioedema, and urticaria (hives) are commonly due to food allergy. Joint pains and arthritis may be food allergy related, as may urinary frequency, hematuria (blood in the urine), and bronchial asthma. Gastrointestinal symptoms are felt by some to be the most common expression of food allergy.

CHAPTER THREE

Specific Foods

MILK

Hippocrates was the first to report allergic symptoms due to milk. Milk is the most common food allergen in America today, probably resulting in more sensitivities than all other foods put together. Pediatricians may be more aware of this than other physicians, but problems adults take to their physicians are due to food allergy more often than they are recognized as such. Constipation is frequently due to milk sensitivity but milk may produce any allergic symptom known. Generalized abdominal pain and distention, which may be diagnosed as mucous or spastic colitis may be due to milk sensitivity.

Milk allergy often runs in families, but may produce different symptoms in different family members. One may have stomachache, another headache, a third asthma, and so on. More than half have more than one symptom (31) and different organs may be involved in separate exposures.

Milk may induce congestion of the nose and bronchial tree, leading to the expression that milk produces phlegm. The large amounts of mucus may be associated with a sore throat.

Frederick Speer, M.D. of the Speer Allergy Clinic, states that milk is almost always a factor in serous otitis media, an infection of the middle ear. Such symptoms as bedwetting, asthma, headache, diarrhea, bad breath, tension, fatigue, and excessive sweating may be traced to milk sensitivity.

People who are allergic to cow's milk are frequently also allergic to goat's milk as well as to beef. Some authorities feel that children given cow's milk at an early age may develop other allergies more readily, including wheat sensitivity. Others report similar proteins in cow's milk and wheat. (30) Several researchers have observed less cow's milk allergy in children who were not given cow's milk for at least six months after birth. Breast feeding decreases the incidence of cow's milk allergy, but breast-fed infants may react to milk consumed by the mother. Some 15 to 20 percent of children allergic to cow's milk are also allergic to soy. (29)

Tests for food allergy are frequently inaccurate, and tests for milk allergy are no exception. Skin testing may be positive in patients who develop skin symptoms from milk, but negative in the patient who develops gastrointestinal, respiratory or systemic symptoms. (29) Cow's milk allergy is often of a delayed reaction type, making it difficult for the patient to associate milk use with his symptoms. Not all unpleasant reactions to foods are allergies; some sensitivities are not dependent on any kind of antigen-antibody reaction and will not be discovered with tests that are dependent on that kind of reaction.

Lactose intolerance may be quite separate from cow's milk allergy, and after a negative lactose intolerance test many physicians rule out the possibility of cow's milk allergy.

A person who reacts to milk may actually be allergic to substances such as penicillin in the milk.

Milk allergy may be worse in the winter, making recognition even more difficult, as it may be confused with colds.

When parents are advised to take their child off cow's milk they often immediately ask "But where will he get his calcium?" Many authorities feel that children who are milk-sensitive do not absorb calcium well from milk anyway, so for them milk is not a good source of calcium. Greens are high in calcium and will supply adequate amounts of calcium for the average person.

MILK-FREE DIET

Elimination is the only way to control milk sensitization; desensitization has been shown ineffective.

The person sensitive to milk will need to be a careful label reader. Traces of milk products are found in a wide variety of foods. Even "non-dairy" products often contain caseinate, a milk protein. Three milk proteins, lactalbumin, lactoglobulin, and caseine are responsible for milk allergy, but lactalbumin is the most frequent. Caseine, lactose, caseinate, sodium caseinate, lactalbumin, curds or whey are all milk products, and foods containing these products must be eliminated.

It may require several months for the full benefit of the milk-free diet to become apparent. Therefore, persons having symptoms that are suspect should plan a six month period of cutting out (not just cutting down) milk and all milk products.

SYMPTOMS OF COW'S MILK ALLERGY

Dermatological
Acne
Angioedema (swollen lips)
Dark circles around eyes
Eczema
Urticaria (hives)

Gastrointestinal
Abdominal distention
Abdominal pain or stomachache
Colic in infants
Colitis
Constipation
Diarrhea
Gas
Heartburn
Indigestion
Intestinal obstruction in infants
Malabsorption
Mouth ulcers
Peptic ulcers
Poor appetite
Rectal bleeding
Vomiting

Respiratory
Asthma
Bronchitis
Cough
Croup
Frequent colds
Hair loss
Nasal congestion
Nose bleeds
Otitis media (earache)
Pneumonia, recurrent
Postnasal drip
Rhinitis/Rhinorrhea (runny nose)
Sinusitis
Sore throat
Stuffy nose
Wheezing

Miscellaneous
Allergic conjunctivitis (red eyes)
Anaphylaxis
Anemia
Arthritis-like symptoms
Bad breath
Bedwetting
Behavioral disorders
Cardiac irregularities
Cor pulmonale (right heart failure)
Cystitis
Failure to thrive
Fatigue
"Growing pains"
Headache
Heart disease
Hyperactivity
Irritability
Lassitude
Leukorrhea (vaginal discharge)
Migraine
Musculoskeletal discomfort
Nephrotic syndrome
Pallor or paleness
Polyarthritis
Sweating, excessive
Tension
Thrombocytopenia

FOODS TO AVOID ON A MILK-FREE DIET

Milk in all forms, including evaporated, dried, or skimmed
Whey
Cottage cheese and other cheeses (including pizza)
Eggs, escalloped, scrambled, omelettes, souffles
Cocoa containing milk solids, all chocolate in any form, Ovaltine, malted milk
Creamed, scalloped or au gratin foods, creamed soups, sauces and gravies
Yogurt, junket, blanc manges
Ice cream, sherbet
Hollandaise sauce, salad dressings
All cola drinks
Puddings, custards
Commercially prepared bakery products, including breads, pancakes, waffles, crackers, doughnuts, soda crackers, zwieback
Prepared flour mixes
Butter, margarine
Caramels, fondant, nougat
Hot dogs, processed meats, hamburger, hash. Many commercially prepared meats, poultry, fish and seafoods contain milk.
Mashed potatoes
Beef – People allergic to milk are generally allergic to beef.

FOODS ACCEPTABLE ON A MILK-FREE DIET

Vegetables
Fruits and fruit juices
Soy milk
Peach or pear juice, apricot nectar, or stewed fruit may be used on cereal in place of milk
Milk-free carob (some bars contain milk)
Ry-Krisp, Triscuits
Vegetable oils
Popcorn made with vegetable oils, or oil-free
Nuts
Olives
Peanut butter

CHOCOLATE AND COLA

Both of these are members of the kola nut family and a person allergic to one is allergic to the other. Cola is found in many soft drinks, and chocolate in cakes, pies, cookies, doughnuts, candies, icings, milk beverages, and some liquid medications.

In addition to the adverse effects of chocolate itself, many people react to the high levels of sugar contained in chocolate, and to the many companion foods such as milk and nuts, as well as to the additives it contains.

SYMPTOMS OF ALLERGY TO CHOCOLATE

Headache, hives (urticaria), asthma, gastrointestinal allergy, eczema and perennial nasal allergy are often due to these foods. Chocolate allergy may produce lesions of the throat and palate which are identical to herpes simplex lesions. (39)

Karaya gum, often labeled "vegetable gum," contains chocolate.

CORN

Corn (maize) allergy may produce the most bizarre manifestations of any allergy. It is found in one of many forms in a wide variety of commercially prepared foods. Corn syrup is found in almost all chewing gum and candy, processed meats such as luncheon ham, sausages, bologna, and wieners, many baked goods, jellies, jams, canned fruits and fruit juices, sweetened cereals, ice cream and pancake syrup. Corn syrup is more likely than other forms of corn to produce symptoms, and fresh corn the least likely. Dextrose (glucose) is corn syrup. (34) Fructose, sorbitol, dextrin and dextrimaltose are made of corn. Unless sugar specifies beet or cane sugar it may be corn-based.

Cornstarch is frequently used to thicken pies and soups, and milk cartons and some cardboard containers are powdered with cornstarch. (26) Corn flour is found in some baked goods. Cracker Jack, hominy, tortillas, Fritos, burritos, enchiladas, tamales, cereals and grits all contain whole corn, as do corn on the cob, canned corn, and popcorn. Corn oil may be used in some mayonnaise, salad dressings and in food preparations, but is expensive and soybean is more often used. Many alcoholic beverages including most American beer, Canadian whiskey, corn whiskey, and bourbon whiskey contain corn. Mush, scrapple, fish sticks, and waffle and pancake mixes often contain cornmeal.

SYMPTOMS OF CORN ALLERGY

Suspect corn allergy when a person complains of what are frequently considered neurotic symptoms. Migraine, weakness, vague aches, torpor, sleepiness, insomnia, irritability, restlessness, and oversensitivity are common symptoms.

Arrowroot or tapioca may be used to replace cornstarch.

SOURCES OF CORN

Adhesives
Ales
Aspirin and other tablets
Bacon
Baked goods – breads, doughnuts, cakes, cookies, frostings
Baking powder
Bath and body powders
Batters and deep-fat frying mixtures
Bee Pollen
Beets, Harvard
Beer
Beverages, carbonated
Bourbon
Candy
Catsup
Cheese
Chili
Chop Suey
Coffee, Instant
Cough syrup
Cups, paper
Dates, confection
Dentifrices
Dry cereals
Desserts – puddings, custards, cream pies, sherbets
Envelopes
Fats used for frying
Flour, bleached
Fried foods
Fritos
Fruit juices
Fruits, canned and frozen
Gelatin
Glucose-containing products
Gravies
Grits
Gum
Hams, tenderized, cured
Honey
Infant formulas, most
Meats, sausages, bologna, etc.
Milk in cardboard cartons

Monosodium glutamate
Oleomargarine
Pabulum
Paper cups may be coated with cornstarch
Peanut butters, some (the oil added is often corn oil, not peanut oil)
Peas, canned
Popcorn
Preserves
Rice, coated
Salad dressings, French dressing
Salt (Most table salt contains corn sugar. Plain sea salt may be used.)
Sandwich spreads
Sauces
Similac
Starch
Stamps, stickers (glue)
String beans, frozen, canned
Soups, creamed or thickened
Soy bean milks
Sugar, powdered, confectioners
Syrups – Karo, Sweetose
Talcums
Tapes
Teas, instant
Toothpastes, some
Tortillas
Vegetable soups
Vegetables frozen, canned, creamed
Vanilla
Vinegar, distilled
Vitamins, capsules, lozenges, suppositories, tablets
Wheat flour, bleached
Whiskies
Wines, some
Zest

EGG

Because egg contains so much protein it is often a potent allergen. Susceptible persons may suffer allergic symptoms after smelling egg! Albumin is felt to be the offending agent in eggs, but yolk may also cause problems. Vitellin, ovovitellein, livetin, ovomucin, ovomucoid and albumin are all egg.

Eggs are found in most baked goods, French toast, icings, meringue, candies, mayonnaise, creamy salad dressings, noodles, meat loaf, and breaded foods. Many vaccines are grown on chick or egg embryo, making them dangerous to the egg-sensitive person. Children allergic to egg are frequently allergic to chicken.

SYMPTOMS OF EGG ALLERGY

Egg is one of the most common causes of infantile eczema. (65) Urticaria (hives), angioedema (swelling of the skin), asthma, headache, and gastrointestinal symptoms are common manifestations of egg allergy.

Many commercially available egg substitutes contain highly allergenic substances and may only trade one set of symptoms for another. An equal amount of mashed banana may be substituted to replace egg as a binding substance in cakes. Extra flour or cornstarch may be used to replace the thickening action of egg in creamed dishes and sauces. In most recipes one tablespoon of vegetable oil and two teaspoons of water will replace an egg. For further information on egg substitutes see SUE'S KITCHEN.

EGG-FREE DIET

Eggs are found in so many commercially prepared foods that one must read package labels carefully to avoid them.

Baked, creamed, scrambled, deviled, fried, boiled eggs, eggnogs, omelettes, sauces and meringues

Cake flour

Salad dressing, hollandaise, and tartar sauce

Breads, breaded foods, French toast, fritters, muffins, waffles, griddle cakes, doughnuts

Baking powder

Cakes, puddings, sherbets, ice cream, custards, Bavarian creams, sponge and angel cakes, macaroons, pie fillings, whips, frostings, blanc manges, candies

Coffee (some are clarified with egg products), root beer, wine, cocoa drinks. Any prepared drink may contain egg constituents

Chicken, meats, poultry, sea food, fish and game

Canned soups

Frying batters

Ice cream, ices

Hamburger mix, meat loaf, patties

Macaroni, noodles, pretzels, spaghetti

Marshmallows

LEGUMES

The pea family is an important source of food allergens and includes peanuts, soybeans, lentils, garbanzos, alfalfa and bean sprouts, guar (gum) and licorice. Mature or dry peas and beans are more likely to induce symptoms than are green or string beans and green peas. Because honey often comes from members of the legume family individuals allergic to legumes may also be allergic to honey.

Soybean oil and concentrate are often found in baked goods, meats, and a wide variety of manufactured foods. Karaya, acacia or arabic and tragacanth are natural gums which are known to produce allergic reactions in some people. These substances are found in candies, ice creams, gelatin products, salad dressings, diabetic foods, toothpastes and tooth powders. Remember that everything introduced into the mouth must be carefully considered when treating food allergy.

SYMPTOMS OF LEGUME ALLERGY

Headache, asthma, hives (urticaria), and swollen upper lip (angioedema) are frequently produced by legumes.

FOODS TO AVOID ON A SOY-FREE DIET

Soy-based milks, formulas, coffee substitutes
Bakery products, including pastries, cakes and rolls, which contain soy flour or oil
Soy is frequently used as an extender in commercially prepared meats.
Pork link sausage and lunch meats may contain soy
Noodles, macaroni, and spaghetti made from soy
Many canned soups contain soy
Cheese substitutes such as tofu, natto, and miso
Soy sauce, teriyaki sauce, LaChoy sauce
Some ice creams contain soy products
Margarine and butter substitutes, Crisco, Spry, Wesson oil and other shortenings. Some mayonnaise and salad dressings contain soy oil.
Lecithin, which is made from soy, is often found in chocolate. Hard candies, fudge, caramels, and nut candies may all contain soy
Soybean sprouts
Foods fried in soy oil (corn chips, potato chips, etc.)
Tuna, sardines, etc. packed in soy oil

ACCEPTABLE FOODS

All fruits and fruit juices
All vegetables
Potatoes, rice

CITRUS

Orange, grapefruit, tangerine, lemon, lime and kumquat are all members of the citrus family. Patients who are allergic to citric acid may also react to pineapple and all tart artificial drinks. Citric acid may come from pineapples, lemons, corn or beet molasses.

SYMPTOMS OF CITRUS ALLERGY

Asthma, eczema, hives (urticaria), and canker sores (aphthous stomatitis) are common symptoms of allergy to citrus. Migraine headaches are often a result of citrus sensitivity.

Sesame flour, which is used as a binder in meat products, cakes, and breads may contain pulverized orange peel. Homemade mayonnaise and whipped toppings, pumpkin or potato pie, all desserts, and salad dressings may contain lemon juice or lemon peel.

TOMATO

Tomato is found in pizza, catsup, soups, stews, chili, salads, tomato paste and juice, meat loaf, and many commercially prepared foods. It may produce asthma, eczema, hives (urticaria), and canker sores, and sometimes headache.

SMALL GRAINS

Probably because of the large quantities of bread and other wheat products consumed, wheat is the most common offender in this family, but barley, rice, oats, millet, rye, and wild rice may also produce symptoms. Wheat is closely related to rice. (34) Rye is felt to be the least allergenic grain in the family, but buying rye bread is not the solution to a wheat allergy as commercially prepared rye bread contains more wheat than rye flour. Buckwheat is a good substitute for wheat, but cannot be used to make yeast raised breads.

Wheat is found in almost all baked goods, macaroni, noodles, and spaghetti, cream sauces, gravies, pie crust, breaded foods, pretzels, cereals, and chili.

Gluten is the main protein found in wheat, and is believed to be responsible for most of the reactions to it. Some foods marked "wheat-free" contain gluten. Starches, stabilizers, emulsifiers, and hydrolyzed vegetable protein are usually wheat-based. (31)

Malt and cereal extracts may contain gluten. Cake, pastry, all-purpose, white bread, self-rising, wheat, whole wheat, cracked wheat, graham and enriched flours all contain wheat, as do wheat germ, semolina, farina, bread crumbs, cracker meal, and self-rising corn meal.

Rice wafers and Ry-Krisp are generally wheat free and are readily available.

SYMPTOMS OF ALLERGY TO SMALL GRAINS

Respiratory, bladder, skin, nasal, nervous and gastrointestinal symptoms are frequent symptoms due to wheat allergy. Gluten allergy may lead to calcium loss, inducing osteoporosis and bone fractures.

Crohn's disease, a chronic, severe inflammatory disease of the bowel may respond dramatically to a rigorous gluten-free diet. Cases of Crohn's disease are reported to be so sensitive to gluten that a single beer will cause a reactivation of the disease.

Cow's milk allergy may cause wheat (gluten) intolerance in later life, which may involve celiac disease. (66, 67) Celiac disease is a syndrome of the small bowel involving malabsorption of gluten and fats. Diarrhea, weight loss, and multiple deficiencies result; it may become life-threatening if not recognized. Some adults with celiac disease are able to tolerate gluten, but not milk. (68) Not giving an infant cow's milk will decrease his likelihood of allergies in later life. Cow's milk is the ideal food – for calves. Human milk is the ideal milk for humans.

WHEAT FLOUR SUBSTITUTES

These substitutes require a longer (10-20 minutes) and slower baking process than does wheat flour. Combine substitutes for a better baked product. Combinations should be well sifted to assure thorough mixing. Small loaves permit thorough baking. Remember that yeast leavening depends on the gluten in wheat, and that breads not using wheat must be unleavened types. See SUE'S KITCHEN for recipes for "quick breads" not using leavening agents.

APPROXIMATE REPLACEMENTS IN RECIPES

For 1 tablespoon of wheat flour substitute:
  1/2 T. cornstarch
  1/2 T. potato starch
  1/2 T. arrowroot starch
  1 T. arrowroot
  1/2 T. rice flour
  2 t. quick-cooking tapioca
  1 T. oatmeal
  1/2 t. sago
For 1 cup of wheat flour substitute:
  1/2 cup barley flour
  1 cup corn flour
  3/4 cup plain bolted cornmeal, coarse
  1 scant cup plain bolted cornmeal, fine
  5/8 cup potato flour
  3/4 to 1 cup rice flour

1 1/4 cup rye flour
1 cup rye meal
3/4 cup oats
1 1/3 cup ground rolled oats
1/2 cup arrowroot flour
1/2 cup cornstarch
3/4 cup potato meal
3/4 cup soybean flour
1/2 cup potato flour and 1/2 cup rye flour
1/3 cup potato flour and 2/3 cup rye flour
5/8 cup rice flour and 1/3 cup rye flour
1 cup soy flour and 1/4 cup potato starch flour

FOODS TO AVOID ON WHEAT-FREE DIET

Postum, Ovaltine, cocoa, malt, malted milk, beer, ale, gin, whiskies

Wheat breads and crackers, rolls, muffins, biscuits, commercially prepared cornmeal muffins; corn bread, spoon bread mixes, pancakes, griddle cakes, waffles made with batter, graham bread, sweet rolls, pretzels, popovers, zwieback, pastries, self-rising cornmeal, degermed yellow corn meal. Any bread which has nicely risen should be considered to contain wheat.

Matzos

Wheat cereals, shredded wheat, puffed wheat, farina, bran

Wheat germ

Breaded meats, fish and meat patties, commercially prepared meats such as cold cuts, wieners, bologna, liverwurst, luncheon meats, hamburger, chili con carne, frankfurters, sausages, commercially prepared stews. Game, meats, poultry, fish and seafood are often prepared with wheat products.

Stuffing for poultry and game, Swiss steaks, and croquettes often contain wheat. Spaghetti, noodles, macaroni, dumplings, stuffing

All cream soups thickened with flour; all canned and instant soups

Cakes, pies, doughnuts, ice cream cones, bread pudding. A wheat filler is often found in commercial sherbets and ice cream. Commercial candies often contain wheat products

Mayonnaise, salad dressings, and gravy thickened with flour

Chocolate and other candy bars may contain wheat starch or malt

Vegetables prepared with sauce

Some baking powders contain wheat

Flours – corn, gluten, graham, white, whole wheat

Bouillon cubes

ACCEPTABLE FOODS ON A WHEAT-FREE DIET

Ry-Krisp, rice wafers, plain bolted corn meal, buckwheat, 100 percent rye
    bread. People who are not extremely sensitive to wheat may tolerate
    very dry Melba toast.
Rice, corn, or oat cereal without malt
Potatoes, rice
Homemade soups
Vegetable oils
Popcorn, tapioca
All fruits
Vegetables prepared without sauces, flour, bread or bread crumbs
Flours – buckwheat, lima bean, rice, barley, oat, and rye

SPICES AND CONDIMENTS

Cinnamon is probably the most potent allergen in this group and is
found in apple pies and other apple dishes, cinnamon rolls, catsup, chewing gum, cookies, candy, chili and many prepared meats. People who are
allergic to cinnamon are generally sensitive to bay leaf as well.

SYMPTOMS OF ALLERGY TO SPICES

Hives (urticaria), headache, and asthma are frequent symptoms of
cinnamon allergy.
Vinegar may produce acute gastrointestinal tract symptoms. (65)
Pepper (black and white), cumin, sage, thyme, spearmint, peppermint,
and oregano may also produce allergic reactions.

SUGAR

Sugar may cause or worsen a variety of allergic symptoms. However,
because sugar is used in such large amounts and often on a daily basis it
is often unsuspected. Sugar allergy (addiction) is very common.
Sugar is processed from corn, cane, or beets. People sensitive to
these foods may react to sugar. Gases used in sugar processing are troublesome to some people.
Sugar also fuels the growth of yeasts (see chapter on Candida) which
produce a large range of human diseases.

COFFEE, TEA, COLAS

Some researchers in the field of allergies believe that a person must
give up caffeine entirely before he can expect relief from symptoms of
food allergy. (59) The use of decaffeinated coffee is often sufficient to
prevent symptom relief. Headache is the commonest symptom we have
found to the "brown beverages."

ARTIFICIAL FOOD COLORS AND FOOD ADDITIVES

Asthma and hives (urticaria) are common symptoms of food color allergy. Yellow dye tartrazine (FD&C Yellow No. 5) and red dye amaranth are the most common offenders. We have recently seen a patient who invariably gets severe joint pains, often lasting one to two weeks, from even small amounts of foods containing Yellow No. 5.

Carbonated beverages, drinks such as Hi-C, and Tang, Kool-Aid, antibiotic syrups, cough syrups and many other medications, bubble gum, popsicles, and gelatin desserts such as jello contain artificial food colors.

We would do well to avoid foods that were processed before reaching the market. Even this will not eliminate insecticides which are sprayed on in the field. Cherries, peaches and apples are sprayed frequently during the growing season. The chemicals sometimes penetrate the pulp, and washing or peeling the fruit is not adequate to remove the insecticides.

Apples, parsnips, rutabagas, cucumbers, green peppers, and squash are often coated with oils to make them shiny. Peeling reduces the exposure.

Commercially dried fruits are treated with sulfur dioxide unless otherwise labeled. Dates which are shipped across state lines are fumigated with methyl bromide, and bananas are often treated with ethylene to hasten ripening. Pears, apples, oranges and tomatoes may also be ethylene-treated. Oranges are frequently dyed. Eggs are sometimes dipped in a penicillin solution to retard spoilage; the penicillin can penetrate the shell and be eaten with the egg. Chickens may be given antibiotics or various other chemicals during their lifetime, which remain in the meat. Killed chickens are sometimes dipped in antibiotic solutions to slow bacterial growth. Fish may be treated in a similar manner before freezing. Frozen potatoes may be treated with sodium EDTA and sodium acid pyrophosphate during processing, and may be coated with methylcellulose to form a crisp crust on frying.

Some people are unable to tolerate foods from cans, but the same product packaged in a glass jar does not bother them. The phenolic resin or plastic liner of the can is felt to be the problem. Others are sensitive to plastic wrap products used to cover foods. Glass is recommended for storing and freezing foods.

WATER

An increasing number of people are having problems with water, most likely due to the chemicals used in purification. Some types of chlorine used in water purification can be removed from water by boiling it for 30 minutes or allowing it to stand uncovered in a glass container for about 12 hours. Other types are concentrated by boiling. A distiller is the most secure way of dealing with water additives. Distilled water may prove troublesome to some if stored in soft plastic containers. If the filters used in home filter systems are made of resins the water may cause a problem. Bottle caps are sometimes plastic lined. (40) Water may be transported in plastic-lined trucks and stored in plastic containers before being bottled in glass, so one cannot be certain that water purchased in glass containers has not been exposed to plastic.

Activated carbon water filters may be very helpful in treating ordinary tap water, but plain charcoal filters are felt by some to be inadequate.

FOOD ADDITIVES

The following additives are known to have induced allergic reactions:

Acacia Gum (Gum arabic) – Candies, chewing gum, glazes, jellies, mustard, pickles, ice cream, skimmed milk, soft drinks, processed cheeses

Almond Flavorings – Same as Vanilla flavoring

Alum – Relishes, pickles, baking powders, starch, flour, liquors, ale

Amaranth Red No. 3 – Breads, dried breakfast foods, snack foods, butter, cheese, fruit juice concentrates, jam, marmalade, ice cream, icing, sugar, liquors, flavored milk drinks, catsup, pickles, smoked fish

Benzoic Acid – Catsup, tomato paste, pickles, relish, pickled fish, jam and marmalade, margarine, miscellaneous flavorings including lemon, chocolate, orange and cherry

Benzoyl Peroxide – Blue cheese, flour

Brilliant Blue FCF – Same as Amaranth, soft drinks, dried drink powders, gelatine desserts, candy, puddings

Brominated Vegetable Oil – Flavored or citrus drinks, soft drinks, ice cream, baked goods, ices

Butylated Hydroxyanisole (BHA) Chewing gum, dried breakfast cereals, dried beverage mixes, dehydrated potatoes, fats, oils, baked goods, gelatin desserts, dry yeast, soup bases, lard

Butylated Hydroxytoluene (BHT) – Fats, oils, dried breakfast cereals, dried beverage mixes, dehydrated potatoes, chewing gum, enriched rice, animal shortenings, frozen fresh pork sausage, freeze-dried meats

Caffeine – Cola drinks, coffee, tea, chocolate, some commercial orange juice, some soft drinks, kola nuts, guarana paste, mate, root beer

Calcium Carbonate – Bread, wine, ice cream, cream syrups, baking powder

Caramel – See Amaranth. Also pickled fish, meats, soft drinks, syrups, confections, baked goods

Carboxymethyl Cellulose – Ice cream, processed cheeses, flavored milk drinks, salad dressings

Citrus Red No. 2 – See Amaranth

Epichlorohydrin – Starch

Erythrosine – Dried breakfast cereals, bread, butter, cheese, fruit juice concentrates, jam, marmalade, ice cream, icing sugar, flavored milk drinks, liquors, smoked fish, catsup, snack foods

Fast Green FCF – Same as Amaranth

Gum Arabic – See Acacia Gum

Indigotin – Snack foods, dried breakfast cereals, bread, butter, jam, marmalade, cheese, fruit juice concentrates, ice cream, icing sugar, flavored milk drinks, liquors, pickles, catsup, smoked fish.

Lemon Flavoring – Same as Vanilla flavoring.

Mineral Oil – Confectionary, coating on fresh fruits and vegetables, vitamin capsules and tablets.

Monosodium Glutamate (MSG) – Canned vegetables, pickles, candy, baked goods, soups, fish and meat. Often found in Chinese foods, and ready-to-eat-foods

1,3-Butylene Glycols – Flavorings

Paraffin Wax – Cheese, fresh fruits and vegetables, chewing gum

Polyoxyethylene Stearate – Bakery products

Polyvinylpyrrolidone – Lager, ale, wine, cider, vinegar

Ponceau SX – Fruit peel, glace fruits and maraschino cherries

Potassium Bisulfite – Ale, beer, wine, tomato puree, lemon juice concentrate, dried fruit, fruit pectin, fruit pie mix

Potassium Metabisulfite – Wine, ale, lemon juice concentrate, tomato puree, dried fruit, fruit pectin

Potassium Nitrate – Ham, luncheon meats, smoked sausage, some cheeses.

Potassium Nitrite – Side bacon, preserved meats and poultry.

Propyl Gallate – Oils, fats, shortening, margarine, chewing gum, dried breakfast cereals, beverages, ice cream, candy, gelatin desserts, baked goods

Propylene Glycol – salt

Saccharin

Salicylates – Bakery goods other than bread, ice cream, candy, chewing gum, soft drinks, jams, gelatin desserts, cake mixes and wintergreen flavored products.

Saponin – Pop, beverage mixes

Shellac – Cake decorations, candies

Sodium Alginate – Baby formulas, frozen fish, coarse salt, ale, malt liquors, lager, flavored milk drinks, cheese, cream, ice cream, mustard.

Sodium Benzoate – Pickled fish, tomato paste, catsup, relish, pickles, jam, and marmalade, margarine, codfish, soft drinks, mincemeat, maraschino cherries, fruit juices, confections

Sodium Bisulfite – Wine, ale, tomato puree, dried fruit, fruit pectin, lemon juice concentrate

Sodium Metabisulphite – Wine, ale, lemon juice concentrate, tomato puree, dried fruit, fruit pectin, sugars, syrups, juices

Sodium Nitrate – some cheeses, smoked sausage, luncheon meats, ham

Sodium Nitrite – Preserved poultry, meats, and side bacon

Sodium Propionate – Breads, cured meats, poultry and fish, cheeses

Sodium Sulfite – cider, wines, beer, dried fruit, canned tuna, biscuit dough, and instant potatoes

Sunset Yellow FCF – see Amaranth, carbonated beverages, gelatin, bakery products, puddings, tablets

Tannic Acid – Chewing gum, wine, cider, honey wine, flavorings

Tartrazine Yellow No. 5. See Amaranth

Tragacanth Gum – Processed cheese, ice cream, skimmed milk, mustard pickles, icings, fruit jelly, fruit sherbets, salad dressings, French dressings, candy

Vanilla Flavoring – Bakery products other than bread, some brands of buttermilk, cocoa, instant soups, pop, powdered fruit drinks, candies, chewing gum, ice cream, medicine, potato chips, ices, puddings, syrups, toppings, ices

MISCELLANEOUS FOODS KNOWN TO CAUSE ALLERGY

Apple*	Cherry	Melons	Rice
Apricot	Chicken	Mushrooms	Sassafras
Arrowroot	Clam	Mustard	Scallop
Artichoke	Cloves	Nuts	Seafood
Banana	Coconut	Okra	Shrimp
Beef	Coffee	Olives	Spinach
Beet	Cranberry	Onions	Squash
Blueberry	Currant	Oyster	Strawberries
Brazil nuts	Fig	Pecans	Sugar
Broccoli	Fish, all kinds	Persimmon	Sweet potato
Brussels sprouts	Garlic	Pineapple	Tapioca
Cabbage	Ginger	Plum	Turkey
Carrot	Gooseberry	Pork	Turnip
Cashew	Grape	Potato, White	Vanilla
Cauliflower	Lettuce	Rabbit	Walnut
Celery	Mango	Rhubarb	Wintergreen

*Some people may be able to eat raw apple if it is peeled.

A person who suspects that he is allergic to a certain food or foods should carefully eliminate them from his diet for three or more weeks. After three weeks, if all symptoms have disappeared, add one food back to the diet, watching for the return of symptoms. Additional foods may be reintroduced at three to seven day intervals.

Eliminating one food at a time may work in the person who is allergic to only one food, but if multiple allergies exist the symptoms will continue, leading the person to believe that they are not due to food sensitivity.

Cooking reduces allergenicity; a person who is sensitive to a food in its raw state may be able to take limited quantities of it after it has been cooked.

CHAPTER FOUR

Diagnosing a Food Allergy

SKIN TESTS

Skin tests involve one of several methods of applying the allergen to the skin. Theoretically the mast cells of the skin release histamine which produces a skin reaction if the person is allergic to the substance. The skin tests are not entirely accurate and can be used only for certain substances. Most food sensitivities are skin test negative; in other words, skin tests are not accurate for diagnosis of food sensitivities.

RAST

Radioallergosorbent testing (RAST) is an ingenious laboratory laboratory test designed to pick up the presence of IgE antibody to a given allergen. However, RAST is unreliable in testing for food allergies. (36) It has been shown to produce approximately 20 percent false positive and 20 percent false negative results. Furthermore, it costs $10 to $12 per test, making it extremely expensive. The typical initial battery of allergy tests checks for about 40 allergens. Initial RAST tests would run more than $400. (56)

BLOOD TESTS

Blood tests may be 25 percent accurate, and are considered unreliable by most food allergists.

PULSE TEST

The pulse test is being used by many allergists. The patient fasts for four to six days, taking only water. After the fast he is given a meal consisting of a single food. His pulse rate is taken before ingestion of the food, and every twenty minutes for one hour after ingestion. Other symptoms are observed at the same time. At each mealtime the process is repeated, using a different food each time. A drop or increase in the pulse of 20 or more beats per minute should be considered significant. Since so many things – from meal companions to the weather – can influence the pulse rate, this test is also not entirely reliable.

ELIMINATION DIET

Since the reaction of the person to a food may involve more than an allergy (an antigen-antibody reaction), and since we have no good laboratory tests for many of the reactions a person may have in response to foods which cause unpleasant symptoms, it has seemed wisest to us to start out with a test on the person in his own environment with the natural usage of the food. We believe this to be the most reliable of the methods attempting to discover food sensitivities. Since there are often both causes and triggers of food sensitivity symptoms, either of which may not be operative at any one time, there may be some detective work needed to make a proper investigation. Several approaches are discussed in this book: the rotary diet, the food diary (trying to correlate symptoms with the eating of certain foods – helpful for occasional symptoms – and the elimination diet (omitting foods until symptoms disappear and reintroducing them one every three to seven days and observing any reactions).

CHAPTER FIVE

Guidelines for the Food Allergy Diet

ROTARY DIET

A rotary diet is a diet in which a food is eaten only one time in every four to seven day period. Marshall Mandell, M.D., feels that a rotary diet carefully followed will in time allow a person to eat 50 to 70 percent of the foods to which he was previously allergic.

To begin a rotary diet make a list of foods you know or suspect you are sensitive to. Eliminate these foods for at least three weeks. This is to allow the allergic symptoms to die down. During the first few weeks eat foods that you have not eaten frequently in the past, as you are unlikely to be sensitive to them.

Make a diet plan for a week, eating only one food per meal. Plan a different food for each of the 21 meals during the week. Do not group together foods in the same food family.

Keep a food diary, listing the foods eaten and time and extent of symptoms you observe. The first week, and sometimes even the second week, will not give a true picture of food sensitivities because symptoms may carry over from foods eaten before the test rotary diet was begun. The diet the second week should be a duplicate of the first week to allow for this phenomenon. Any food which produces symptoms should be eliminated for at least three months.

After a food-induced reaction you should fast until symptoms clear. Some foods felt to infrequently produce allergic symptoms are:

Apricots	Green beans	Raisins
Barley	Kiwi fruit	Rye
Beets	Melons	Spinach
Carrots	Peaches	Squash
Celery	Pineapple	Sweet Potatoes
Cranberries	Plums	Tapioca
Grapes	Prunes	Vanilla extract

FOOD FAMILIES

Study the list of food families below. Avoid selecting many foods from a single family:

Apple – Apple, pear, quince

Aster – Artichoke, chamomile, chicory, dandelion, endive, escarole, lettuce, safflower, sunflower, tarragon

Banana – Banana, plantain

Beech – Beechnut, chestnut, chinquapin nut

Beet – Beet, chard, lamb's quarters, spinach

Blueberry – Blueberry, huckleberry, cranberry

Cashew – Cashews, mango, pistachio

Citrus – Citron, grapefruit, kumquat, lemon, lime, mandarin, orange, tangerine

Grains – Barley, corn, lemongrass, oats, rice, rye, sorghum, verbena, wheat, wild rice

Laurel – Avocado, bay leaf, camphor, cinnamon, sassafras

Legumes – Beans, carob, cocoa, lentils, licorice, lima, mung, navy, pinto, soy and string beans, peanut, black-eyed, chick and green peas, soybeans, tamarind

Lily – Asparagus, chives, garlic, leek, onions

Melon – Cantaloupe, cucumber, honeydew, muskmelon, pumpkin, squash, watermelon, zucchini

Mint – Basil, catnip, horehound, lemon balm, marjoram, mint, peppermint, rosemary, sage, savory, spearmint, thyme

Mulberry – Breadfruit, fig, mulberry

Mustard – Broccoli, Brussels sprouts, cabbage, cauliflower, Chinese cabbage, collards, kale, kohlrabi, mustard, radish, rutabaga, turnips, watercress

Nuts – Brazil nuts, pecans, walnuts

Parsley – Angelica, anise, caraway, carrot, celery, coriander, cumin, dill, fennel, parsley, parsnip

Plum – Almond, apricots, cherries, nectarine, peaches, plums, persimmon, prune, wild cherry

Potato – Eggplant, paprika, peppers, pimiento, potatoes, tomato, tobacco

Rose – Blackberry, boysenberry, dewberry, loganberry, pomegranate, raspberry, rose hip, strawberry

Sunflower (see Aster) – Artichoke, lettuce, sunflower

Walnut – Black walnut, butternuts, English walnuts, hickory nut, pecans

FOOD DIARY

Keep a record of everything you eat for several weeks. Don't try to remember what you have eaten – record it immediately after you eat. List every ingredient in mixed and combination foods. If you eat a sandwich record the dressing and kind of bread.

In another column of your diary record symptoms, using a scale to indicate severity. Mild symptoms may be 1, severe symptoms may rate a 4.

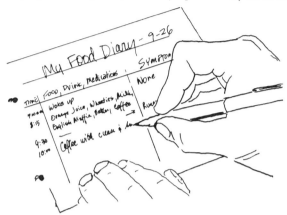

Record any food cravings. List your favorite foods and drinks.

Weigh yourself each morning. A sudden weight gain may indicate fluid retention, a sign of food sensitivity.

A simple, but not always totally accurate way to establish a list of suspect foods is to compare a list of foods eaten on a day you felt well with a list from a day you felt bad. Eliminate foods on both lists, and the foods left on the list for the bad day may be considered suspect. The chief weakness with this technique is that delayed symptoms may be overlooked.

ELIMINATION DIETS

There are several forms of elimination diet, and we will not discuss all of them.

If you already suspect a food or foods, you may eliminate these foods from your diet for three to eight weeks, letting the disappearance of symptoms determine the length. You must be very strict, eliminating the suspect foods in all forms. This does not mean to cut down on the food, but to cut it out. Many people fail in the test because of failure in this point. After three weeks eat one of the foods – in generous amounts. Watch for the return of symptoms. Every three days, add back another suspect food.

Some people have so many allergies it is difficult to trace all of them down. Such a person may may need to go on a total fast, taking nothing but pure water for four or five days. At the end of the fast you may eat a single food per day, observing symptoms. Test a different food each day, keeping a diary of foods and symptoms. Remember that during the fast you may suffer "withdrawal" symptoms, which may make you feel worse, but if the problem is a food allergy, the symptoms will be cleared by the fifth or sixth day. Bear in mind that more than one food may be offending, and when one food is discovered to cause a return of symptoms, do not think your work is finished. Continue to add foods back one every three days.

Drinking adequate quantities of pure water is absolutely essential during the fast period. Distilled water may be used if no other source of pure water is available. Many people are sensitive to chemicals in tap water.

MISCELLANEOUS SUGGESTIONS FOR THE FOOD ALLERGY DIET

Herbs and oils should also be rotated. To keep mixtures to a minimum use corn oil with meals containing corn, soy oil with soybeans, etc. Bear in mind that many people are sensitive to oil and all other free fats.

Use a diet as close to its natural state as possible. Avoid processed, refined, and "junk" foods. Alcohol, caffeine and tobacco should be eliminated.

Use a minimum number of foods at each meal. Many highly allergic people find better symptom relief with only one food per meal, using another food at the next meal to assure variety. Avoid eating the same food more than once a day. The more often a food is eaten the greater likelihood there is of developing an allergy to it. The greater the number of foods in one meal, the greater the likelihood of developing an allergy to something in the meal. Both menus and recipes should be as simple as possible with as few items combined as possible.

Some people find a dietary of only one food per meal quite monotonous and these people may elect to use a combination of two or three foods per meal. The more foods added to a meal the more taxing it is to the body to digest and absorb all the various chemicals which are presented to it.

A person with food allergies must learn to be a careful label reader. Unfortunately, not all ingredients must be listed, and even if listed vague terms may be used. A diet composed of foods in as natural a state as possible will go far toward minimizing these problems.

1. A food reaction may be shortened by the use of a dose of magnesium sulfate (epsom salts) (55), or by charcoal.
2. Use fresh foods whenever possible. Keep the use of processed foods to a minimum. When canned or packaged foods are used read the labels carefully.

3. All processed meats should be eliminated as they may contain a wide variety of allergens. Meat in any form should be suspect because of the likelihood of antibiotics, hormones, etc. that have been given to the animal and may remain in the meat after the animal is slaughtered.

4. Canned fruits packed in syrup should be avoided, as the source of sugar is difficult to determine. Use instead fresh fruits or fruits packed in their own juices.

5. Canned fish may be canned in vegetable oil.

6. Nuts should be purchased in the shell or obtained from a source where one can be certain that they are additive free. Commercially available nuts may be roasted in a dry pan in the oven at 275 degrees.

7. Commercially available peanut butter often contains sugar. Pure peanut butter may be made at home, or obtained in health food stores. See SUE'S KITCHEN for recipes.

8. Use simple foods rather than complex mixtures. Keep each meal simple. Do not combine or mix foods. Use only two or three different foods at a single meal.

9. Sometimes people can tolerate such foods as apple or orange if it is given to them peeled. The skin may provoke symptoms, while the edible portion does not. This applies to both fruit and vegetables.

10. After an allergenic food is eliminated from the diet for a period of three weeks the person may be able to eat it in limited quantities without inducing allergic symptoms. To maintain this status the food should not be eaten more than once a day every four or five days.

11. Sometimes foods not tolerated in the raw state may be eaten cooked.

12. Fermented or decomposed proteins are more likely to produce an allergic reaction than are fresh proteins.

13. People may be allergic to all foods of a certain family without having eaten all of them because of the cross-reactivity or similarity of the allergens.

14. Use as much additive-free food as possible. A person not allergic to a food may be allergic to an additive used in processing. Colorings, flavorings, preservatives, emulsifiers and stabilizers often induce allergic symptoms. Growing your own fruits and vegetables will assure a safe supply. Chemical sprays may induce reactions and lead a person to think he is allergic to the food. There is no reliable test for additive sensitivity.

15. Foods wrapped in plastic wrap or sold in plastic tubs may induce symptoms due to substances they impart to the foods. Foods wrapped in plastic should be aired before they are eaten. Plastic wrapped foods sealed with a wire twist may adequately air in three to four days. To hasten airing you may place the food in a glass jar which contains a charcoal filter. Foods heat-sealed in plastic may never be adequately

aired. Canned foods sometimes absorb chemicals from the can lining.

16. Modified food starch may come from arrowroot, tapioca, wheat, sorghum, corn, or potatoes.

17. Sulfites may not be listed on food labels.

18. Foods from highly allergenic food families should be rotated. Apples and pears are in the same family. If you eat a pear on Monday do not eat an apple until Thursday or Friday.

19. Foods which belong to the same family as foods you know you are allergic to should be eaten sparingly, and on a rotating schedule.

20. Water was felt for many years to be non-allergenic, but some people are now showing reactions to substances, such as chlorine, which have been added to the water. Water may become moldy when stored in bottles. Sterilize bottles and caps from time to time. To sterilize glass jars place them uncapped in the oven at 250 degrees F. for 90 minutes, or boil for 20 minutes.

21. Foods which are known to be highly allergenic (such as milk, eggs, and nuts) should not be used more often than once a week.

22. Use a wide variety of foods in your diet. The greater the variety the less likely you are to develop new allergies to foods.

23. Fats subjected to high temperatures may form allergenic substances. Some allergic persons do best with foods cooked at low temperatures. A diet low in free (added) fats may also be quite helpful.

24. Parents may do much to prevent food allergies in children by breast-feeding the child, and not giving him the same food more than once a week when he starts on solid foods. Dr. Joseph Morgan, an Oregon pediatric allergist, feels that there might be no food allergies if a child were given a rotary diet, without sugar or additives. (70)

25. Commercial yeast may contain corn, rye, or barley. (71) Persons sensitive to corn may use Red Star yeast, which is corn-free.

CHAPTER SIX

Breast Feeding and Food Allergy

Breast feeding has been shown to be effective in decreasing food allergies. The digestive system of newborns is still immature, and the mechanisms that prevent allergic reactions are not fully activated. Breast milk contains minimal amounts of foreign protein. The introduction of solid foods, particularly those which are highly allergenic, should be delayed as long as possible. (40) The more mature the infant's digestive system is at the time of introduction of solid foods the more likely he is to be able to tolerate them. Foods should be introduced in small amounts, one at a time. New foods should not be given more often than once every four days. (43) Give only a bite the first time, increasing the amount with each feeding if no adverse effects are observed.

Rice or oat cereals, mixed with water or breast milk, may be the best solid food to start the infant on. Wheat should not be given to an infant before he is 9 to 12 months of age. Use single foods, not mixtures.

Raw fruit, other than very ripe banana, should not be introduced to the child's diet before 12 months of age. Cooked fruits may be given earlier. Apples, peaches, berries, barely ripe bananas, and citrus fruits should be the last fruits introduced. Pears, plums, and apricots are felt to be low-allergenic.

Carrots, beets, squash, potato and asparagus are vegetables which are generally well tolerated. Beans, spinach, and peas should not be given before the child is 12 months old. Tomato and corn are probably best withheld until the child is two years old.

Cereals should be cooked in water for three or more hours. There is some evidence that poorly cooked grains are responsible for many of the sensitivities we see in adults to small grains such as wheat, corn, rice, and oats. Yeast breads should be cut into finger shaped slices and dried thoroughly and lightly toasted in a 250 degree oven to make melba toast, the most easily digestible of breads.

Because allergies tend to run in families, breast feeding is particularly important for infants whose parents have allergies. The practice of giving cow's milk formula is undoubtedly a contributing factor in the high incidence of cow's milk allergy in America today. Failure to breast-feed is a common source of illness and disability throughout the lifetime of the individual. The intestinal mucosa may be so severely injured by milk consumption that it never recovers, and the person remains allergic to milk throughout his life. Cow's milk appears to increase sensitivity to all types of environmental allergens. (69)

Not only may the infant develop allergy to milk, but he may become sensitive to substances eaten by the cows, and transmitted through the milk. Ragweed in cow feed may lead to hay-fever-like symptoms, bran to a wheat allergy, and peanut hay to peanut allergy. (42)

It has recently been demonstrated that breast-fed infants may have allergic reactions to foods eaten by the mother and transmitted to the infant via the breast milk. Authorities are now recommending that breast feeding mothers avoid such highly allergenic foods as milk, eggs, pork, shellfish, alcoholic beverages and nuts. Milk and eggs are by far the most frequent offenders, but various studies have shown that oranges, apples, bananas, chocolate, coffee, wheat, citrus fruits, corn, rice, legumes, peanuts, beef, strawberries, tomatoes, pork, and onions may all cause problems.

Ten babies who had been totally breast-fed developed eczema which cleared only when their mothers discontinued the use of eggs. Another infant suffering from eczema improved after his mother ceased the use of chocolate, and it returned when she used it again. (41) Others have suffered colic from their mother's intake of milk. Breast-feeding mothers are still eating for two!·

Allergic symptoms generally do not occur at the time of first exposure to a food, but newborns may react to a food the first time it is fed to them. Researchers now understand that the infant may become sensitive to a food which his mother eats during the pregnancy. J. Glaser and Douglas E. Johnstone recommend that mothers avoid the use of dairy products during pregnancy because of the high potential for sensitization, and Johnstone and Arthur M. Dutton suggest the elimination of eggs. (40) If milk and eggs are not eaten by the expectant or nursing mother, care should be taken that whole grains, not refined grains, be taken. If she will eat legumes, greens, and whole grains, the mother can easily replace all the nutrients in milk and eggs, as these are the foods cattle and chickens eat to produce milk and eggs. There should be no skimping on the mother's food. She must have the best quality and adequate quantity of food to supply her needs. Breakfast should always include fruits and whole grains, and lunch should always include vegetables and whole grains. See SUE'S KITCHEN for delicious recipes and menus.

CHAPTER SEVEN

Diseases Which May Be Related to Food Allergy

ABDOMINAL DISTENTION

Abdominal distention or bloating may be a manifestation of food allergy.

ABDOMINAL PAIN

William G. Crook, M.D. states that a food allergy is the most common cause of otherwise unexplained abdominal pain in children. (9) This stomach pain may be accompanied by aching legs and other symptoms of allergy.

Abdominal pain is a common complaint of both allergic and non-allergic persons. Because food-allergy induced pain may involve the whole abdomen and change location from one time to the next the patient is often considered neurotic. If the pain becomes localized it frequently appears in the right side and flank, in one of the upper quadrants (the right most often) or around the umbilicus. (24) It may be misdiagnosed as appendicitis.

ACNE

Food allergies are frequently responsible for acne. Egg, peanuts, nuts, colas, and chocolate have been discovered to induce acne. In our experience milk is frequently responsible for acne, especially when it is combined with sugar and eggs as in breads, snacks, and ice cream products.

ALBUMINURIA (PROTEIN IN THE URINE)

Food allergy is a frequent cause of albuminuria, the commonest form of protein in the urine. Serum protein which appears in the urine after a child has been upright, but disappears when he lies down is called orthostatic albuminuria. A study performed in Japan revealed that many children with albuminuria also showed such symptoms of food allergy as fatigue, nausea, dizziness, weakness, headache, palpitations, etc. Food allergens to milk, eggs or soybeans were found in all patients in this study. (16)

ALLERGIC TENSION-FATIGUE SYNDROME

Dr. F. Speer coined the term "allergic tension-fatigue syndrome" for a set of symptoms which are composed of both fatigue and tension manifestations.

Delayed food allergy is the most common cause of this problem, making it very difficult for patient, family, or physician to trace the cause of the problem. With fatigue symptoms the child feels tired and often weak. He may stop playing in order to sit and rest. He may put his head down on the desk at school and be difficult to arouse in the morning. Symptoms may persist even when the child has had a good night of sleep. Dr. William G. Crook, a leading authority on pediatric allergy, says that in his experience the most common cause of unexplained fatigue in children is allergy.

At the other end of the scale, an allergic child may become hyperactive. He may be constantly in a state of motion, fidgeting, twisting, turning, jumping, and jerking about. These children may be irritable and impossible to please, and often gain the reputation of being spoiled. (9)

ALVEOLITIS (LUNG DISEASE)

Alveolitis, a serious inflammation of the alveoli or air sacs of the lungs may be due to milk allergy. (5) Symptoms include fever, loss of appetite, cough, and feeling very bad.

ANEMIA

Allergy may be the most frequent cause of pallor in the pediatric office. It may be confused with anemia as anemic children also look pale. The pallor of allergy is frequently accompanied by dark shadows under the eyes, often called "allergic shiners." Sensitivity to free fats (margarine, mayonnaise, fried foods, cooking fats) is often a cause of dark circles around the eyes but milk and other food sensitivity may produce the same symptoms. A month or more may be required to remedy the circles, after omitting the offending food.

Infants given milk may develop anemia due to bleeding from the gastrointestinal tract.

ANOREXIA (LOSS OF APPETITE)

Some people who are allergic to milk develop poor appetite. Omitting the milk leads to increased appetite and weight gain. (36) Others allergic to milk have a voracious appetite which is brought under control when milk is eliminated.

ANOREXIA NERVOSA

A Connecticut psychiatrist tested a group of anorexics and found every one of them to have serious abnormalities. Some of these people responded to a program designed to lower exposure to allergens, but much research still remains to be done in this area.

ARTHRITIS

Protein may be the most frequent cause of food sensitivity in arthritis. (17) Pork, milk and milk products (including cheese), corn, wheat, fish, whiskey, beer, lettuce, white potatoes, string beans, chocolate, beef, eggs and chicken have been implicated as producing joint pain.

Arthritis symptoms are late manifestations of food allergy; reactions to pork may not appear for five days after consumption. This makes it very difficult to determine the relationship.

Another very important group of foods causing food-sensitivity arthritis is the nightshade group. This family of plants includes tomatoes, potatoes, tobacco, eggplant, and peppers (paprika, pimientos, etc.).

Dr. Norman Childers, Professor Emeritus of Horticulture at Rutgers University, writing in the *Journal of the International Academy of Preventive Medicine* (72) calls attention to toxic alkaloids in the nightshade family of plants. An arthritic syndrome in cattle has been found to be related to nightshade plants. Interestingly, the active form of vitamin D was demonstrated to be the culprit in these plants. Dr. Childers and others have noted that many arthritics are aggravated by milk, and suspect that the added vitamin D may be responsible. Dr. Childers also points out that solanine, the alkaloid present in potatoes, has cholinesterase-inhibiting properties; that is, in high doses it can block an enzyme essential for proper function of nerves and muscles. Many potent insecticides and pesticides have the same property and muscle stiffness, soreness, and pain have been reported after exposure to them.

At least ten percent of cases of arthritis due to food sensitivity are said to be due to nightshade sensitivity. It is always well worth a trial on a diet totally devoid of nightshades to determine if this is a problem. One 91 year old lady who had been in a wheelchair for eight years due to arthritis had relief of pain in two weeks on a nightshade-free diet. Her stiffness disappeared after four weeks on the nightshade-free diet. She became able to get around without the wheelchair. Sometimes as long as three to six months are required to relieve symptoms. In later communications, Dr. Childers believes that as many as 50 percent of arthritics will obtain significant relief if they adhere strictly to a nightshade-free diet for six months.

Dr. Childers cautions that the diet must be strict; even bits of the nightshades are sufficient to nullify the effect of the diet. Foods listing "natural flavoring" as an ingredient may include nightshades. Some yogurts contain potato starch as a thickener. Some cheeses, particularly the pinkish colored ones may contain paprika. Herbal teas may contain capsicum (pepper). Baby foods may contain potato and tomato products. A simple diet, free from commercially prepared foods, will decrease the possibility of unknowingly consuming nightshades. Dr. Childers also reports that chocolate, vitamin C supplements, cortisone or gold shots, tea and coffee may may also cause problems.

Fluid accumulation in the joints may be responsible for the symptoms. This fluid accumulation is temporary, but permanent changes may eventually occur if the offending food is not eliminated from the diet.

A 38-year old woman with an 11 year history of rheumatoid arthritis reported feeling better with decreased morning stiffness three weeks after eliminating milk and milk products from her diet. After 10 months she ate cheese and symptoms returned. She has since remained on her diet and is fully mobile and was able to discontinue the use of Prednisone. (25)

ASTHMA

Milk, seafood, chocolate, peanut, fish, corn, nuts, wheat, onion, and garlic allergies are frequently responsible for asthmatic attacks. Other foods may also be involved in some persons with asthma.

BAD BREATH

Unpleasant or bad breath is a common but often unrecognized symptom of food allergy. The patient may report that if he eats a certain food he tastes it all day. Milk, eggs, and chocolate are the most common offenders. (54)

BEDWETTING

Allergy is often the cause of bedwetting in children. When these children eat a food to which they are sensitive, it produces spasm of the smooth muscle in the urinary bladder, making the bladder contract. The contracted bladder is unable to hold as much urine and the child often urinates more frequently during the day, and wets the bed at night.

James C. Breneman, M.D. observed that there was a family or personal history of allergy or allergic symptoms present in every patient he was treating for bedwetting. A group of 60 children troubled with bedwetting were studied for food sensitivities; the suspected offending foods were removed from their diet. Every one of the children ceased bedwetting within three to seven days. (11) As soon as the bedwetting stopped the allergy could be confirmed by adding back a food every two to three days. When a food causes bedwetting it is removed from the diet for one year. Then the confirmation test is repeated by giving a small portion of the food to which the child had been allergic to see if the allergy has disappeared. Dr. Breneman found milk, citrus fruit, egg, chocolate, and some cereal grains to be the most frequent food sensitivities causing bedwetting. (12)

BRONCHIAL ASTHMA AND RHINITIS

Over 300 children with rhinitis and/or bronchial asthma were placed on an elimination diet to evaluate the possibility of food allergy as a factor in the disease. As is often the case in asthma, previous allergy tests performed had been negative. Of the 322 children, 91 percent showed significant improvement (61 percent had almost complete clearing of symptoms), and 30 percent showed some improvement. Only 9 percent had no significant improvement. Milk, egg, chocolate, soy, legumes, and corn were the symptom-producing foods in this study, but other studies list milk, chocolate, citrus, legumes, corn, eggs, and tomatoes as common allergens. It is estimated that 20 percent of infants allergic to cow's milk are also allergic to soy products. (4) Our young patients with asthma are often responsive to an elimination diet. The easiest way to handle the diet is to remove at one time all the foods on the list of common allergens for a month or two, until the symptoms are clear or very nearly so. Then begin adding foods back to the diet, one at a time, every three days until symptoms reappear. Stay off the foods causing symptoms for one year to allow time for recovery from the allergy.

BRUXISM (TEETH GRINDING)

There are three times as many cases of bruxism reported in allergic as in non-allergic children. (46)

BURSITIS

Bursitis may be induced or worsened by allergic reactions.

CANKER SORES (APHTHOUS STOMATITIS)

Gastrointestinal symptoms often accompany mouth ulcers or canker sores, suggesting that food allergy is the most common precipitant of mouth ulcers. Citrus, apple, chocolate, spices (particularly cinnamon), coffee, nuts, and caraway are felt to be the most frequent offenders.

CELIAC DISEASE

Celiac disease has been associated with intolerance to gluten, but some patients must also exclude soybeans. Some people will not have relief of celiac symptoms until eggs (38) or milk are omitted from the diet. The gluten intolerance may be induced by early exposure to cow's milk, resulting in permanent damage to the intestinal tract.

CEREBRAL PALSY

Many victims of cerebral palsy suffer an increase in the intensity of their symptoms because of allergies. Recognizing and removing these allergens may improve their quality of life. (57)

COLIC

Colic in breast-fed infants may be due to the mother's intake of cow's milk. Studies suggest that a macromolecular substance in cow's milk is transmitted to the baby through the breast milk, and produces colic. Eliminating cow's milk from the mother's diet results in prompt disappearance of the infant's colic. (45)

COLITIS

Milk is the most frequent cause of colitis. (17) Egg, chocolate, meat, nuts, wheat, corn, and citrus have been documented as causes of colitis. Complete elimination of dairy products has resulted in remissions in chronic ulcerative colitis.

CONSTIPATION

Constipation is sometimes produced by food sensitivity. Milk is most often the offending agent, but chocolate and many other foods – different for each person – may also produce constipation. The foods may set off spasms in the bowel which interfere with the normal elimination.

COORDINATION, LACK OF

Incoordination or clumsiness is one of the more distressing symptoms caused by allergy. (23) These individuals are subject to frequent falls, are unsteady on the feet, and act clumsy at times.

CROHN'S DISEASE

Crohn's disease, or regional ileitis, a very severe and disabling inflammatory disease of the bowel, may respond dramatically to a gluten-free diet (gluten is the main protein in wheat, but is also found in small quantities in oats, barley and rye). Gluten restriction must be rigorous.

One professor of gastroenterology said that he had seen flare-ups from drinking one beer, the malt being the culprit in that case.

One 30-year-old woman was seen who had had a large segment of bowel removed, was very ill with constant and painful diarrhea and bleeding from Crohn's disease. She was on a large dose of cortisone and had cortisone-induced diabetes, with 40 units of insulin not controlling her blood sugar. After two weeks on a gluten-free diet and simple hydrotherapy, she was free of pain, bleeding, and diarrhea. She has been able to stop cortisone and insulin, with blood sugars entirely normal. She subsequently graduated from college and is working productively.

CROUP

Recurrent croup may be due to food allergy. (36) Before considering the use of pharmaceuticals always try a hypoallergenic routine – food restriction, warm extremities, exercise, sunshine, plenty of water, and a relaxed mental attitude.

CYSTITIS

Young girls who suffer from recurrent bouts of cystitis may be suffering a food sensitivity. Milk is the most common allergen, but eggs, chocolate, cereal grains, citrus fruit, food colorings, black pepper, tomatoes or other foods may be the problem. (54)

DEAFNESS

Difficulty hearing may be due to sensitivities. Tobacco smoke is known to produce blockage of the eustachian tube, postnasal drip, and symptoms of sinusitis. Fluid retention in the hearing structures may result in impaired hearing. (58)

DIABETES

Diabetics with food allergy may suffer from elevated blood sugar, making diabetic control much more difficult. Some may even manifest insulin resistance. (17)

DIARRHEA

Food allergy is often accompanied by diarrhea. Allergen elimination is effective in controlling the problem. Milk and sugar are probably the most common offenders. Lactose-intolerance, present in large numbers of the population is responsible for many cases of gas, abdominal pain, and diarrhea. Abstinence from dairy products should always be tried in these cases.

DIZZINESS

Dizziness may be due to allergy, but dizziness is frequently caused by other factors. If another cause cannot be found an allergy study may be worthwhile.

DUODENAL ULCER, CHRONIC

James Breneman states that chronic duodenal ulcer is frequently produced by a gastrointestinal allergy to milk. (17) Patients given milk, the longstanding treatment for ulcers, do not heal permanently, but rather develop into a persistent and chronic problem. Especially when the person does not chew food to a cream, and does not drink sufficient water between meals to maintain tissues in a state of excellent hydration both day and night, the problem of food sensitivities is intensified.

DYSMENORRHEA

Some patients have reported relief of painful menstruation after they eliminated foods to which they were sensitive. (65) The problem is known to be related to constipation and irritability of the gastrointestinal tract, and any food sensitivity could easily interfere with motility of the genital organs by reflexive action, or cause pelvic congestion due to blockage of blood vessels in constipation.

ECZEMA

Cow's milk allergy is the most common cause of eczema in infancy. The milk can be taken by the infant, or by the mother of a breastfeeding infant. When the milk or other offending foods are removed from the diet, several weeks may be required for the eczema to clear. During that time the child should be washed in pure water, no soap, dried with towels washed only in water, and lightly covered with vaseline milk made by blending vaseline and water half and half in a blender to make a thick emulsion about like mayonnaise, and lightly smoothing on the child's skin. It will need to be stirred often to remix water and vaseline. Keep it in the refrigerator as it will spoil. When drying the skin, blot dry with a towel rather than rubbing as rubbing opens microscopic cracks that make the eczema continue.

EDEMA

Fluid retention may be caused by food sensitivity. This may be of such low grade that it is frequently not recognized. There may be puffy eyes. Sensitivity to salt and oil are often the cause of this kind of symptom.

EPILEPSY

A 19-year-old girl treated unsuccessfully for epilepsy stopped having seizures when beef was eliminated from her diet, according to Dr. John Crayton, an associate professor of psychiatry at the University of Chicago Medical School.

During the 1920's and 1930's a number of cases of allergy-induced epilepsy were reported in the medical literature. Foods are the most frequent allergens responsible for convulsive reactions. Milk, eggs, wheat, chocolate, beef, pork, veal, and cheese are the foods most commonly implicated, but others may be involved. Careful detective work may be required to discover the problem food or foods.

Susan C. Dees, M.D. and Hans Lowenbach, M.D. reported in *Modern Medicine* for December 1, 1951 on 37 children who had either petit or grand mal seizures. All symptoms of allergy, as well as seizures, were controlled when the foods to which they were allergic were removed from their diet. The symptoms returned when the children were challenged with the eliminated foods.

FATIGUE

Fatigue is often due to food allergy. This fatigue may actually be worsened by rest, and is often worse in the morning or after naps. It is likely that far more people suffer allergic fatigue than we are aware. Children who complain of fatigue should be studied for allergies. Chronic dehydration is usually a part of the picture, but is difficult to spot. The person may drink water, but because of food sensitivities may be storing it in the tissues or putting out excessive quantities in the urine. The person with fatigue should drink extra water, eat raw vegetables and fruits generously, and use all concentrated foods very sparingly.

FEVER, LOW GRADE

A fever of 99 to 99.8 degrees F. which is otherwise unexplained may be due to food allergy. (20)

GALLBLADDER DISEASE

J. C. Breneman placed a group of patients felt to have gallbladder disease on a basic elimination diet. While on the diet all of them had complete relief of their symptoms. Adding eggs back into the diet produced gallbladder symptoms in 83 percent of the patients in the study. Foods in the categories of pork, onion, milk, coffee, fowl, orange, corn, beans, nuts, apple, tomato, peas, cabbage, spices, peanut, fish and rye produced symptoms in smaller percentages of patients.

The many patients who continue to have food intolerances after gallbladder removal may be simply continuing to exhibit food allergies, the cause of their symptoms all along. Symptoms may be due to edema of the bile ducts, irritability of the structures of the biliary tree, or direct irritation of the ducts outside the liver, including the duodenum into which bile empties.

GOUT

Food reactions affect gouty arthritis. Gout patients who have been shown to be sensitive to certain foods improved when those foods were eliminated.

HAY FEVER

The person with allergic rhinitis, who suffers stuffy nose, sneezing, runny nose, itching eyes and nose and tearing may be suffering from food allergy, or it may be complicating inhaled allergens such as dusts, molds and pollens. A number of cases have reported that eliminating milk, eggs, and chocolate brings considerable relief. If a person has frequent "colds" he should check for food sensitivities as an irritation initiated by a food can weaken the tissues sufficiently to allow the invasion by a virus or bacterium.

Puffiness and wrinkling around the eyes, known as "Denny's Sign," is sometimes associated with hay fever.

HEADACHES

Many children who complain of headaches are suffering food allergies. It is felt that the foods produce an allergic reaction which causes spasm and other changes in the blood vessels inside the head. Fluid may leak out of these vessels and the brain may swell, causing headache, pain, or throbbing. (9)

HIGH BLOOD PRESSURE

Dr. Lloyd Rosenvold of Idaho was probably the first to observe a relationship between high blood pressure and allergies. He observed that when some of his patients ate foods they were allergic to they suffered an increase in blood pressure levels. A Sacramento, California physician reported lowered blood pressures in all of a group of people who eliminated from their diet foods to which they were allergic. A London neurologist, Dr. Ellen Gant, observed a similar response when she placed a group of hypertensives on a diet free of the foods known to induce migraine. Pork is also known to elevate blood pressure in sensitive individuals.

HIVES (URTICARIA)

Hives are frequently produced in response to the intake of egg, peanut, chocolate, preservatives, spices, flavoring and coloring agents.

HYPERACTIVITY

Dr. Benjamin Feingold, a San Francisco allergist and pediatrician pointed out the relationship between allergy and hyperactivity. He eliminated salicylate-containing foods (almonds, apples, apricots, blackberries, cherries, cloves, cucumbers (including pickles), currants, gooseberries, grapes and raisins, mint, nectarines, oranges, peaches, plums, prunes, raspberries, strawberries, tomato, aspirin and wintergreen) with good success in many children. Unfortunately, the fact that the diet did not work for all children caused a number of medical people to reject it. Dr. William G. Crook, a Jackson, Tennessee pediatrician points out that such foods as sugar, eggs, milk, chocolate, citrus fruit, corn and wheat may produce the same symptoms in children sensitive to them. Dr. Crook says that sometimes three weeks on the diet may be required before the child demonstrates relief of symptoms. Younger children tend to respond more quickly than do older ones or adults. Yes, adults do suffer from hyperactivity. It often goes by the name of "highstrung" in adults.

HYPOGLYCEMIC SYNDROME

Persons suffering from the hypoglycemic syndrome have been observed to have large increases or decreases in their blood sugar levels after eating foods to which they were sensitive. We believe that much of what passes in the minds of patients as "hypoglycemia" is actually a food sensitivity, particularly in persons having strange thoughts, phobias, depression, compulsions, or mental illness.

INSOMNIA

Insomnia, dating to early childhood, often accompanies food allergy. Sometimes the patient falls asleep normally, but awakens in the early morning hours, remaining awake for several hours. This may be a delayed reaction to foods eaten several hours previously.

ITCHING

Itchy skin may be due to allergy. Histamine (released into the skin during an allergic reaction) irritates the nerve endings of the skin.

LEARNING PROBLEMS

Food allergy may play an important role in the development of both behavior and learning problems in children. A child who is stuffy, drowsy, suffering headache or stomachache will not be able to perform well in school. Dr. William Crook feels that allergy is the most important cause of learning problems in many children. (9) He did a study which revealed that 41 of 45 children with learning difficulties were relieved totally or partially of their symptoms when put on a diet free of the foods they were allergic to. They demonstrated the ability to learn with clearing of the allergy symptoms. (9) A study conducted by Jerome Vogel, M.D., medical director of the New York Institute for Child-Development suggests that over 75 percent of children with learning disabilities have allergies. He feels that refined sugar is the main offender.

We recall a 14 year old patient who had been tested and found to be of normal intelligence, whose mother was at her wits end because of incessant misbehavior, destructiveness, and maladjustment in the home, the church, and his school. He had never made passing marks in school and was a trial in every way. He had been given barbiturates and amphetamines at different times by other physicians, largely without any change except to make him a goody-goody who continued maladjusted and unpleasant to supervise. Within a month of simplifying his homelife, removing television and radio, and making radical changes in his diet, he became a model son – obedient, non-aggressive, studious and friendly with other students.

MENIERE'S DISEASE

Thirteen out of fourteen Meniere's patients evaluated were found to be allergic to either inhalants or foods. (1)

George E. Shambaugh, Jr, M.D., Professor Emeritus of the Department of Otolaryngology of Northwestern University Medical School in Chicago reports that his symptoms were relieved after he learned that he should avoid milk, wheat, coffee, yeast, and house dust to which he was allergic. He says that when he was an infant his mother often walked the floor with him screaming with colic. As a child he craved milk, even imagining a faucet on his bed that he could turn on to obtain milk day or night. He states that colic is a prime symptom of milk allergy. Food addiction or cravings are frequently symptoms of food allergy. (6)

A 49-year-old woman with symptoms of Meniere's disease over a five-year period had complete relief of all her symptoms with a diet free of milk, pork, and eggs, and a low salt intake. After a two year period she resumed the eliminated foods and developed a sensation of pressure in her right ear and partial loss of hearing. Dr. Lewis Dahl's guidelines for taking a diet with less than 1000 mg. of salt daily (used for his blood pressure patients) is as follows: 1) add no salt to food, at the stove or at the table, 2) Use no dairy products as they are naturally high in salt. Mammary glands are related to sweat glands, and excrete a lot of salt. 3) Use no processed foods (meats, baked goods, spreads, sauces, canned foods and some frozen), 4) Use no salted foods (nuts, chips, etc.)

A 54-year-old female suffered loss of hearing, pressure, ringing in her ears and vertigo (dizziness), headaches and colitis for four and a half years. Tests revealed that she was allergic to yeast, eggs, chicken, corn, chocolate and tomatoes. The dizziness, colitis, and headaches were completely cleared with omission of the offending foods, and her hearing, sensation of pressure, and ringing in the ears improved.

A 56-year-old lawyer had symptoms of dizziness, partial loss of hearing, and irritability which required four tranquilizers a day. Elimination of wheat, citrus fruits, yeast, eggs and coffee improved his symptoms to the point that he could discontinue the use of tranquilizers.

After suffering with Meniere's disease for 12 years a 40-year-old woman was discovered to be allergic to milk and wheat. The dizziness, ringing in the ears, and hearing loss improved when she eliminated these foods from her diet. Two years later the dizziness returned. Repeat tests revealed that she was sensitive to yeast, eggs, milk, coffee, onion, pineapple, orange, grapefruit and wheat. When these foods were eliminated she reported feeling better than at any time previously. (6)

Dr. Shambaugh cautions that not every person with Meniere's disease has food allergies, but many do. He also points out that the more frequently a food is eaten, the more likely it is that there is an allergy to, and a craving for it.

MENOPAUSAL SYMPTOMS

Several reports suggest that menopausal flushing or sweating may be caused by or worsened by allergies. Allergic reactions may suppress estrogen production. Allergic reactions can suppress the respiratory center in the brain, causing under breathing, accumulation of heat and sudden breaking out in a sweat, similar to the production of "night sweats" in respiratory disorders.

MIGRAINE

Migraine in adults may be caused by inhalants, but childhood migraine is typically due to food sensitivity. The child often has stomachache at the same time of complaining with headache. As the child matures there is less likelihood of having the stomachache with the headache, but the headaches often become more intense. (9)

Sixty migraine patients placed on an elimination diet had a very dramatic improvement in their migraine headaches: eighty-five percent became free of headaches. One-quarter of the patients who had high blood pressure demonstrated normal blood pressure after a month on the program. Common foods causing migraines in this group of patients were wheat, orange, egg, tea and coffee, chocolate, milk, beef, corn, cane sugar, and yeast. (10)

MONONUCLEOSIS

A "pseudomononucleosis" with enlargement of the cervical lymph glands and fatigue may be due to food allergy. Because this condition often occurs in high school and college age students it may be considered mononucleosis. Dr. Crook reports that he treated about twelve of these students with an allergen-free diet, completely eliminating their unusual fatigue. (9)

MUSCULOSKELETAL SYMPTOMS

A frequently overlooked cause of musculoskeletal pain is allergy, according to several researchers. Intermittent joint swelling due to food allergy was first described about 50 years ago.

Theron G. Randolph, M.D. states that food allergy is the most common cause of allergy-based musculoskeletal symptoms. If a food is suspect it should be eliminated from the diet for a week, then tested. Musculoskeletal manifestations of allergy may not appear for 12 to 36 hours after consumption of the food. Dr. Frederick Speer observed that nearly all patients with extensive food allergies suffer muscle aches.

Allergic muscle aches appear most commonly at night and may be intense. Often the muscles used the most are affected. Dr. Speer states that "there can be no doubt that many of the traditional 'growing pains' of childhood are due to allergy." (15)

Physicians seeing a child with food-induced musculoskeletal symptoms may suspect rheumatic fever or nervousness. The fact that nervousness often accompanies these symptoms supports that theory.

A ten year old girl was seen with complaints of leg pains which developed shortly after she went to bed at night and sometimes interrupted her sleep. She had a history of nasal stuffiness and asthma over the previous five years. Two or three days after the elimination of citrus fruit her muscle aches disappeared. (14)

A 12 year-old boy who had complained of painful knees for six months, had to be taken out of school because of intense pain. He had developed fatigue, irritability, lassitude, headaches and rhinitis after the onset of the muscle pains. His family history was strongly positive for allergies. He was found to be allergic to corn, chocolate, potatoes and peanuts. His pains disappeared with the elimination of these foods, and he became more happy and energetic.

While allergic children frequently suffer "growing pains" women may complain of neck, shoulder, and arm pain brought on by household duties and men may have pain in the arms and back if they are engaged in heavy work.

NASAL POLYPS

L. M. Barsocchini, formerly Assistant Clinical Professor, Department of Otolaryngology, at the University of California at San Francisco, states that he has found food to be responsible for more cases of nasal polyps than any other factor. (3) Nasal polyps are always benign, and are caused by chronic swelling of the lining of the nose, almost always due to allergies.

NEPHROSIS

Nephrosis (a kidney condition with swelling and loss of protein in the urine) may be worsened by the intake of food allergens. Six children with nephrosis were found to worsen after the use of foods to which they were sensitive. Drugs are often involved in worsening nephrosis. Overeating and too much protein also put a tax on the kidneys and can cause the condition to worsen.

NAUSEA

Repeated bouts of nausea may be due to food allergy.

OBESITY

Sensations of hunger or thirst may be an allergic reaction. Weight control is easier when allergens are eliminated. The hypoglycemic syndrome with low blood sugar often follows the intake of allergens. The reactions to the allergen, plus a craving (addiction) for that which is injuring one, as well as the low blood sugar, sets off an almost uncontrollable hunger, leading to weight gain from frequent eating.

OTITIS MEDIA

Otitis media, an inflammation of the middle ear, (earache) is more frequent in bottle-fed than breast-fed infants. Many authorities feel that cow's milk allergy produces inflammation and blockage of the infant's eustachian tubes which lead to infection in the middle ear. Others feel that Immune globulin A present in breast milk strengthens the infant's immune system.

A 1977 study revealed that the majority of children with recurrent otitis media had allergies. (1) Milk, egg, and wheat products are often responsible for fluid in the middle ear. (3) Robert J. Dockhorn, M.D., Associate Professor of Pediatrics at the University of Missouri-Kansas City School of Medicine and Chief of the Allergy-Immunology Section of Children's Mercy Hospital, Kansas City, Missouri, states that in serous otitis media a single allergen is seldom responsible for the sensitivity, but a single food may be the responsible agent, and milk is the most likely allergen. (5) In some people milk will cause mucoid otitis media only during grass season. (3)

POST-NASAL DRIP

Post-nasal drip may be due to allergy. Spicy foods, in particular, are known to produce this allergic symptom.

PRURITUS ANI (ANAL ITCHING)

Food allergy is the most common cause of pruritus ani. Milk, coffee, tea, colas, beer, chocolate, tomatoes, black pepper, and citrus fruits are the most common foods involved.

RESTLESS LEG SYNDROME

Allergic patients often have restless leg syndrome. (22) This syndrome is the cause of much sleeplessness, therefore sleeplessness and food sensitivities sometimes go together. Coffee has been, in our experience, the most common food offender in restless legs, but many other foods can also be at fault.

SALIVATION

Excessive saliva production is sometimes indicative of food allergy.

SENSORY OVERREACTIVITY

Allergic people are often abnormally sensitive to noise and may hold their hands over their ears to eliminate noises that are not disturbing to others.

They may overreact to skin stimuli, finding any type of touch annoying. They may be extremely ticklish.

Odors may be unusually troublesome to allergic persons, being troubled by odors unnoticed by others about them. It is interesting to observe that persons with schizophrenia also often have heightened sensory perception and irritability.

SINUSITIS

L. M. Barsocchini, formerly Assistant Clinical Professor of the Department of Otolaryngology at the University of San Francisco feels that over 40 percent of all cases of sinusitis are allergic in nature and have no causative bacterial factor. (3) Certainly, bacteria and viruses are not the primary factor in most cases, but the food sensitivity came first, and the germ second.

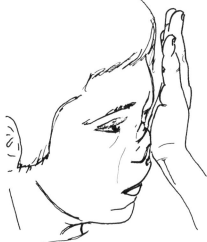

"Allergic Salute." An attempt to clear chronically clogged nasal passages.

STUTTERING

Mild forms of stuttering may be due to food allergy. (21) Milk has proven to be the culprit in some cases.

SWEATING, EXCESSIVE (HYPERHIDROSIS)

Allergic children often exhibit excessive sweating. The sweating may be most prominent about the head of an infant, and the chest of an older child. This sign can be helpful in diagnosing food sensitivities in babies and children.

TEARS (LACRIMATION)

Tearing is not uncommon in allergic individuals, particularly children.

THROMBOPHLEBITIS

Ten patients with recurrent episodes of thrombophlebitis were tested for allergies. Eight of the ten had recurrence of phlebitis during allergy testing. During a five-year follow-up there were two cases of phlebitis among the treated patients while there were 101 episodes in the control group not tested for allergies. (18)

TINNITUS

Ringing, roaring, or crackling noises in the ears may be due to food allergies. Milk, eggs, and wheat have been implicated as causes. In our experience with tinnitus sugar, honey, and other sweeteners have been the most frequently found causes. This problem is often difficult to fully eliminate, and quieting rather than total elimination of the head noise may be acceptable. Some persons find a softly played cassette player to be helpful in getting to sleep at night – the time when tinnitus is most annoying.

ULCERS

Milk, typically given to treat ulcers, may instead produce continuation of symptoms, due to allergic reaction. Dr. James C. Breneman put a man with a ten year history of duodenal ulcer on an elimination diet free of milk, eggs, and wheat. The man had complete relief of his symptoms within three days. Symptoms returned when he used milk again. He was later discovered to be allergic to pork and wheat. Dr. Breneman followed the man for 16 years with no return of the ulcer symptoms. It has been pointed out that the bland diet given for ulcers may be helpful because it eliminates many allergenic foods.

UPPER RESPIRATORY TRACT INFECTIONS

Chronic or recurrent upper respiratory tract infections may be indirectly due to food allergy. The nasal and sinus membranes become swollen, opening the way for the entrance of microorganisms. Milk, egg, corn, wheat, spices, citrus fruit, coffee and chocolate have all been found to be frequent offenders. Tonsils and adenoids which are in the area may also be involved in the inflammatory process.

URINARY TRACT INFECTIONS

Allergy may be the cause of frequent urinary tract infections in children. A 1957 study evaluated 114 patients with recurrent urinary tract infections. Every one of them showed manifestations of allergy. (13) All but one of 57 patients in another study had noticeable improvement in symptoms of urinary tract disease when steps were taken to control their allergies.

Tomatoes, citrus fruit, chocolate, seafoods, condiments, eggs, milk, and wheat are common offenders. Allergic hematuria has been described by several authors.

VAGINAL DISCHARGE

Allergy may cause vaginal discharge. Foods, especially food additives and colorings, and bubble baths and soaps may be responsible for these symptoms. (9)

VAGINITIS

Vaginitis may be due to milk or pollen allergy. (59) Itching and burning may also be due to a local sensitivity to skin bacteria. A cold or hot water pour done each time the bathroom is used day or night, will abolish many cases of vaginitis with itching. Simply pour a full cup of hot or cold water (not lukewarm) through the pubic hair and allow it to run over the vaginal area. Blot dry with tissue.

VERTIGO

Vertigo may be due to an inner ear allergy. See discussion above on Meniere's disease.

VOMITING

Vomiting is a common sign of food allergy in infants; in adults and older children it is not frequently seen.

CHAPTER EIGHT

Food Allergies and the Mind

Some physicians feel that 60 to 70 percent of symptoms considered psychosomatic are due to undiagnosed allergies. (62) Even small amounts of allergenic substances may be involved in many psychological illnesses. (51) Depression, inability to concentrate, anxiety, hostility, and confusion may result from exposure to these substances.

Dr. Ben Feingold pointed out the relationship between food allergies and hyperactivity in children. Other researchers have demonstrated other behavioral changes in allergic children. Nervous behavior, which has resulted in psychiatric treatment, has been often exhibited. (52) Many adults treated for years by psychiatrists have cleared in a month after eliminating foods to which they are sensitive.

Allergic children may demonstrate an unusual sensitivity to pain and/or chilling which is part of a sensory over-reactivity. This exaggerated response to the environment may produce sleep difficulties.

Physical incoordination has been demonstrated in allergic children.

Psychological tests reveal that allergic children manifest more symptoms of anxiety than do non-allergic children.

W. W. Duke observes that mental problems in allergic people are quite common. (53) A. J. Rowe observed mental confusion, lack of initiative, drowsiness, despondency. and lack of energy. W. C. Alvarez in 1946 reported a woman who suffered extreme anxiety after the use of milk. T. W. Clarke reported extreme excitement, destructiveness, and hyperactivity due to allergy. Feelings of unreality, anxiety, inability to concentrate, impulsiveness, depression and hot temper due to allergy were reported in a 1952 paper. Frederic Speer in 1958 reported delirium or severe excitement due to a wheat allergy.

MENTAL SYMPTOMS SOMETIMES RELATED TO FOOD ALLERGY (53)

Agitation
Anxiety
Compulsions
Concentration, lack of
Confusion
Consideration of suicide
Crying easily
Cruelty
Delirium
Delusion
Depression
Difficult to please
Disorientation
Distraction
Dreaminess
Drowsiness
Easily hurt
Erratic
Excitability
Fearful
Feelings of unreality
Hallucinations
"High-strung"
Hysteria
Impatience
Insomnia
Irresponsibility
Irritability
Jumpiness
Lethargy
Loss of interest in life
Mania
Meanness
Mental confusion
Morbidness
Nervousness
Neuroses
Nightmares
Panic
Paranoia
Psychoses
Pugnaciousness
Quarrelsomeness
Rage
Restlessness
Screaming
Sensitiveness
Slow thought processes
Stupor
Talkativeness
Temper
Tenseness
Uncooperativeness
Unhappiness
Unpredictableness
Unreasonableness
Whining
Worries

AGGRESSION

Aggression has been known for years to be sometimes due to allergy. It is suspected that the brain swells, just as the skin sometimes becomes swollen in an allergic reaction. This swelling may produce personality changes such as aggression. Kenneth E. Moyer, Ph.D., professor of psychology at Carnegie-Mellon University says that milk, chocolate, cola, corn, and eggs are the most likely foods to trigger this type of allergic reaction. Low serum glucose has been associated with aggressive behavior.

ALCOHOLISM

Some allergists feel that food allergies play a role in alcoholism. A group of alcoholics tested for allergies showed nearly twice as many allergies as a comparable group of non-alcoholics. Like others who develop cravings for foods they are allergic to, alcoholics crave these items. A person sensitive to yeast, sugar, or grapes may drink wine; the person who drinks rum may be craving sugar cane and a person sensitive to corn, yeast, sugar, or malt may drink beer or bourbon.

Alcohol also worsens other allergic manifestations.

ANXIETY

Allergic persons show significantly greater levels of anxiety than do non-allergic people. When people have unexplained or unjustified anxieties it is worth a trial of food elimination to determine if foods are the culprit. Coffee is frequently an anxiety producer. All forms of caffeine (coffee, tea, cola, chocolate, several soft drinks, some orange juice preparations and caffeine-containing medications) should be eliminated. Nor can one rest assured that the decaffeinated beverages will be tolerated, as the caffeine is by no means the only substance in these items causing sensitivities.

DEPRESSION

Depression, particularly if associated with other symptoms of allergy may be due to food allergy. This relationship was first reported by Dr. Theron Randolph as early as 1950. Dr. Randolph reports life-long cases of depression which cleared with allergen elimination. (59)

Serotonin, a neurotransmitter, which appears to help maintain a positive mental outlook, is made by the body from tryptophan. A diet low in tryptophan may reduce serotonin levels, inducing depression. Corn is low in tryptophan and it is very common in the American diet in many hidden forms. A single meal may significantly influence serotonin levels. (63)

HYPOCHONDRIA

It is probable that many people with obscure and undiagnosable complaints who are labeled hypochondriac are actually suffering from a food allergy, according to Claude A. Frazier, M.D., a prominent Asheville, North Carolina allergist. (8)

IRRITABILITY

Sugar, milk, food coloring, eggs, chocolate, or corn sensitivity may be the cause of irritability.

PSYCHOTIC EPISODES

Food allergy may produce edema (swelling) of certain areas of the brain, which can change the personality, reflexes, and motor activity, or the function of the central nervous system.

SCHIZOPHRENIA

During times of war, with decreased food supplies, it was noted that there was a decrease in admissions of schizophrenics to mental hospitals. This led curious researchers to study the effects of food upon schizophrenia. Two groups of schizophrenics admitted to a psychiatric ward and placed on different diets revealed that those placed on the cereal-free, milk-free diet improved more quickly and were discharged from the hospital in half the time of the group given the standard diet. (48) It was determined that gluten was the troublesome factor.

Schizophrenia is rare in areas of the world where little or no cereal grains are used, and more frequent in countries where wheat, rye, or barley are commonly used.

Another interesting observation was that many patients with celiac disease also have psychiatric symptoms. When the gluten-free diet brought improvement in the celiac symptoms, the mental problems also improved. (49)

Milk protein appears to enhance the effect of wheat gluten in some celiacs. (50)

A 1982 study reported that 80 percent of schizophrenics in one study were allergic to eggs. (60) Caffeine may worsen symptoms of schizophrenia. (61)

VIOLENT AND CRIMINAL BEHAVIOR

The large amount of sugar consumed in the typical American diet may be responsible for a large amount of the violent behavior observed today. The pancreas is overworked in response to the large amount of sugar used (the average American consumes over 129 pounds per year). About 70 percent of our sugar intake comes from the highly processed and refined foods we eat, and since we do not add this sugar ourselves we are often unaware of how much we actually consume. The high sugar intake overworks the pancreas, resulting in overreaction and subsequent low blood sugar. When sugar is in short supply the area of the brain responsible for the thought processes goes into a sort of hibernation, to provide more glucose for the part of the brain that has to do with aggression and defense.

Alcohol has a similar effect on the body, but in a more marked degree. A Loma Linda University study revealed that feeding rats large amounts of sugar created a craving for alcohol.

Many schizophrenics are hypoglycemic, as are people with various other psychiatric problems.

Alexander Schauss reported in his book, DIET, CRIME AND DELINQUENCY, that chronic male juvenile offenders consumed an average of 64 ounces of milk daily, while a control group of non-offenders drank only 30 ounces daily. Delinquent females used an average of 35 ounces of milk a day, while non-offenders used only 17 ounces per day. This may be just the beginning of our understanding of the influence of food allergens on crime rates.

CHAPTER NINE

Candida Albicans and Allergy

Candida albicans (pronounced can' di duh) is a yeast organism found in the gastrointestinal and genitourinary tract, and skin of everyone. It is felt to enter the newborn during birth or shortly thereafter. By six months of age 90 percent of infants have positive skin tests to Candida. By adulthood everyone is felt to harbor this yeast. The immune system normally keeps it in check, but some weakening factors, particularly drugs, sometimes allow the overgrowth of the yeast. The person may become chronically ill, and be completely unaware that Candida is the cause of his illness. Candida may play a major role in worsening food sensitivities.

Birth control pills upset the body's chemistry, sometimes permitting Candidal (pronounced can' di dul) growth. Even the biochemical changes that occur in women during the menstrual cycle are sufficient in susceptible women to stimulate the growth of Candida. Many antibiotics such as tetracycline, ampicillin, erythromycin, keflex and amoxicillin kill the good bacteria in the intestine, allowing unchecked growth of the yeast. Cortisone, prednisone and other immunosuppressant drugs so weaken the immune system that the body is unable to control growth of the yeast. Any symptoms which begin shortly after a vaccination or during or just after an illness in which antibiotics have been taken are suggestive of Candidal infection.

Diet also plays a role in Candidal infection. A person who eats a lot of chocolate, sweets, and other highly refined carbohydrates, dairy products, and many fruits provides just the fuel Candida thrives on.

As the yeast grows and multiplies a variety of toxic products are released in the bloodstream. These toxins overwhelm the immune system, which is in turn unable to control the yeast growth, creating what can become a vicious cycle. All the time the sufferer may be unaware that he even has a yeast infection.

PROBLEMS WHICH MAY BE DUE TO CANDIDA OVERGROWTH

Abdominal distention and bloating
Acne
Agitation
Anxiety
Arthritis
Asthma
Bladder infections
Chemical allergies
Cold hands and feet
Colitis
Concentration, Lack of
Confusion
Constipation
Cramps
Cystitis, recurrent
Depression
Diarrhea
Earaches
Endometriosis
Fatigue
Food allergies
Food cravings
Gas
Gastritis
Hairiness in females
  (when not hereditary)
Hay fever
Headaches
Heartburn
Hives
Hostility
Hyperactivity
Hyperirritability
Joint stiffness and aches
Kidney infections, recurrent
Lethargy
Memory loss
Menstrual problems
Migraines
Movements, uncontrolled
Muscle aches and pains
Numbness, tingling
Schizophrenia
Sinusitis
Skin rashes
Thrush
Ulcer-like symptoms
Urethritis
Vaginitis

A Birmingham, Alabama allergist, Dr. Orian Truss, has done the major research on chronic Candidal infections and their relationship to human disease. He reports that patients with multiple sensitivities are the most likely to be suffering from this yeast infection. A person who has one or two sensitivities is less likely to respond to his treatment routine.

Diagnosis of Candida albicans infections is very difficult; there is no specific test for it since nearly everyone reacts to the skin test. It may be notoriously difficult to grow on culture. Sometimes the best diagnostic procedure is to treat the patient and observe response. The lifestyle of the patient, if carefully examined, can give the alert observer more information as to the likelihood of this type of infection than can any diagnostic test currently in use.

Improvement may be apparent within a few weeks of the start of treatment, or it may require two or three years of treatment to see satisfactory results. Patience and persistence are essential.

Dr. Truss' program for chronic Candidal infection includes the following:

1. Avoid antibiotics, birth control pills and cortisone types of drugs including Prednisone.

2. Avoid high-mold environments.

3. Use a low-carbohydrate diet. Yeast colonies thrive on carbohydrates. Use a carbohydrate counter to lower your carbohydrate intake to 60 to 80 grams per day. The person may actually crave carbohydrate foods and these cravings must be mastered.

4. Limit the use of all yeast foods and their near relatives:

    Baked goods containing baker's yeast

    Foods enriched with vitamins (often made from brewer's yeast)

    B-vitamins (There are some all rice bran B-vitamins)

    Vinegars

    Mushrooms

    Fermented foods and beverages such as sauerkraut, ginger ale, root beer, alcoholic beverages

    Foods containing molds – sour cream, yogurt, buttermilk, all kinds of cheeses

    Malted products

    Dried fruit

    Citrus juice, unless you have squeezed it yourself

    Citric acid and monosodium glutamate are often yeast derivatives.

Other helpful measures include eating foods which inhibit Candida growth (broccoli, garlic, onions, turnips, kale, cabbage).

Woodburning stoves and fireplaces may contribute to the problem as almost all wood contains fungi.

Clean all fresh foods carefully to remove chemicals, sprays, bacteria and fungi. Insecticides, cologne and tobacco should all be avoided, as should any other chemical pollutant.

Reduce mold and dampness in the home.

Nystatin is frequently given to kill off the yeast infection, but some people are bothered by the colored coatings. A powder is available which can be mixed in water. One-eighth teaspoon of powder equals one tablet, and Dr. Truss gives one tablet four times a day after meals. After three to six weeks if improvement is not apparent, Dr. Truss increases the dosage to two tablets four times a day. The suspension preparation of nystatin is sucrose based and the suppositories are lactose based, so neither of these preparations are advisable. Both sucrose and lactose feed the yeast, therefore sweetened foods and foods containing milk or milk derivatives must be avoided. Garlic has been demonstrated effective against Candida, and we recommend its use rather than the Nystatin usually used by Dr. Truss. Nystatin, another antimicrobial, may prove, as have so many other pharmaceuticals, to merely change the location and expression of disease. It is precisely this that Dr. Truss is postulating in the initiation of Candida infections – the use of antibiotics, cortisone and Prednisone, and birth control pills. Additionally, nystatin is extremely expensive whereas dehydrated garlic tablets, (not garlic oil capsules, since many contain only minute quantities of garlic oil in fillers of other vegetable oils) are less expensive. Arizona Natural Products makes a consistently high quality garlic tablet. Garlic and parsley can be obtained in one tablet which seems to help eliminate the garlic odor. Actually, the garlic odor is usually dissipated within a few minutes of taking the tablets. One should start with four tablets twice a day, increasing to eight tablets twice a day if necessary after two weeks.

Some of the experts in Candidal therapy allow no fruits at all in the diet. We hesitate to restrict fruits entirely, but in severe cases we have eliminated fruits for up to two months with benefit. In this case the person eats mostly whole grains, breads made without yeast, vegetables of all kinds, legumes (beans) of all kinds and salads made with raw vegetables. Ripe olives (salt packed, not vinegar), and avocado may be eaten freely. We have not seen a problem in the use of some nuts.

After two months, fruits may be cautiously re-introduced. It may be advisable to avoid the sweeter ones, such as bananas, dates, raisins and other dried fruits, for a prolonged period.

Some of the newer anti-candidal therapies include the use of Caprystatin and/or Lactobacillus acidophilus. Caprystatin is a preparation of caprylic acid, an eight-carbon organic acid found in butter. It is known to be fungistatic in moderate doses and fungicidal in larger doses. Since it is absorbed and digested in the small bowel, it has been considered useless for the treatment of candida. However, the problem seems to have been overcome by combining it with an ion-exchange resin, which is said to deliver the caprylic acid intact to the colon, where it attacks the yeast organisms on the surface of the bowel. A dosage of six tablets a day is recommended. A solution for use in a vaginal douche is available.

Lactobacillus acidophilus is a normal constituent of the colon, but may be in short supply in heavy meat eaters and in those who have taken potent antibiotics. The rationale for using lactobacilli is that its growth will help to "crowd out" and check the growth of Candida in the bowel. Its use has suffered from a lack of potent preparations and often a short shelf life. Several new products now claim to have eliminated these problems by introducing very high potency preparations which have a shelf life of six months or more when refrigerated. A dosage of one-half teaspoon in water three times a day is recommended. A cautionary note is that some of the new preparations contain minute traces of milk products from the culture media. Representatives of the companies marketing them have assured us that reactions to the milk are extremely rare; however, if milk allergy is known or suspected, caution is advised, starting out with no more than one-fourth teaspoon a day.

Both of these products are available in many large health food stores. We have used them in a very limited way so far. It is too early to draw any clearcut conclusions as to their efficacy. We can say that so far we have seen no adverse reactions, and that results in some cases appear guardedly optimistic.

The treatment of chronic Candidiasis requires patience, perseverance, and careful attention to details. Often several weeks are required before results are seen, and sometimes treatment must be continued for several months. Dr. Truss has some cases who have required years of treatment. We believe that treatment to be as effective without Nystatin as with it as both our method and his require a long period of time for recovery.

With the wide publicity being given to this condition, and frequent vagueness of symptoms, there is a real danger that every psychosomatic symptom will be attributed to Candida and the patient may flit from one anti-candidal routine to another in a vain effort to obtain relief. We have seen several such patients, many of whom need life-style changes primarily. Dr. Truss has cautioned against this problem, insisting on the typical history of recurrent yeast infections, exposures to antibiotics, hormones, or corticosteroids along with the symptom complexes typical of the disorder. Multiple, nearly intractable allergies and irritable bowel syndrome are most commonly seen. If these criteria are followed, persistent treatment may be rewarded by dramatic improvements or cures in otherwise baffling or intractable conditions. Much research is currently being carried out by Truss and associates at the University of Alabama and in other cities. Certain "markers" in the immune systems of these patients are now being identified with increasing consistency, and the time may not be too far distant when we shall see fairly easily obtained and clear-cut diagnostic tests. Meanwhile, the search for better and simpler treatment routines goes on.

Allergen – something which produces an allergic reaction.

Allergy – reaction to a substance normally considered harmless.

Anaphylaxis – shock, excessive sensitivity to a substance.

Angioedema – swelling of the skin due to an allergic reaction, usually the upper lip and eyelids. Usually appears suddenly and regresses just as suddenly.

Anorexia nervosa – prolonged loss of appetite

Antibodies – substances produced by the body in response to an antigen

Antigen – A substance which stimulates production of an antibody

Aphasia – inability to speak

Aphthous stomatitis – canker sores

Atopic – allergic

Bursitis – inflammation of a bursa

Candida albicans – a yeast-like fungus

Canker sores – mouth ulcers

Celiac disease – a disease of sensitivity to gluten and atrophy of the upper small intestinal mucosa. Symptoms include diarrhea, malnutrition, and nutritional deficiencies.

Colitis – inflammation of the colon

Conjunctivitis – red eyes, inflammation of the conjunctivae

Cor pulmonale – right heart failure

Crohn's disease – an inflammatory disease of the bowel

Croup – a respiratory problem marked by cough and difficulty breathing

Cystitis – inflammation of the bladder

Eczema – an inflammation of the skin, often characterized by itching, redness, and oozing lesions

Endometriosis – the presence of functioning endometrial tissue in locations where it is not normally found

Gastritis – inflammation of the lining of the stomach

Gout – painful inflammation of joints

Hematuria – blood in the urine

Hypochondria – abnormal obsession with one's health, often with imaginary physical problems

Hypoglycemic syndrome – low blood sugar, also called premature aging syndrome

Immune system – the body system which protects against infection

Lactose – milk sugar

Lassitude – fatigue, weakness, listlessness

Lethargy – indifference, laziness, drowsiness

Leukorrhea – a white discharge caused by inflammation or congestion of the mucous membranes of the vagina

Lymphocytes – a type of blood cell produced by lymphoid tissue; a type of leukocyte

Melancholia – extreme depression

Mononucleosis – a disease characterized by fever, feeling bad, sore throat often, and an increase of certain white blood cells in the blood

Mucous membrane – lining of a moist surface such as the mouth

Osteoporosis – a decrease in bone density

Otitis media – earache, inflammation of the middle ear

Palpitations – abnormally strong heart beats, often with increase in frequency

Peritonitis – inflammation of the peritoneum

Pugnaciousness – belligerent, eager to fight

RAST – Radioallergosorbent testing. A test for antibodies usually unreliable in testing for food allergies

Rhinitis – inflammation of the mucous membranes of the nose

Rhinorrhea – runny nose

Thrombocytopenia – reduction in number of blood platelets

Torpor – sluggishness, dullness, apathy

Urethritis – inflammation of the tube leading to the outside from the urinary bladder

Urticaria – hives of the skin, frequently accompanied by burning and itching

Vaginitis – inflammation of the vagina

Vertigo – dizziness

BIBLIOGRAPHY

1. Pediatrics 50:346, 1972

2. American Journal of Otology 3(4)379-383, April, 1982

3. Primary Care 9(2)371-383, June, 1982

4. Annals of Allergy 44:273-278, May, 1980

5. Otolaryngolic Clinics of North America 10(1)103-12, February, 1977

6. Otolaryngolic Clinics of North America 13(4)671-679, November, 1980

7. Laryngoscope 87:1650-1657, 1977

8. Behavioral Medicine, June, 1978 p. 10-13

9. Pediatric Clinics of North America 22(1)227-238, February, 1975

10. The Lancet 1:966, 1979

11. GP 20:84, 1959

12. Family Practice News, April 1, 1980, p. 6

13. Annals of Allergy 28:252-255, June, 1970

14. Int. Arch Allergy 14:84, 1959

15. Int. Arch Allergy 12:207-214, 1958

16. Journal of Asthma Research 3:325-329, 1966

17. Breneman, J. C. MD Basics of Food Allergy. Springfield: C. C. Thomas, 1978

18. Annals of Allergy 47:338-344, November, 1981

19. Int. Arch. Allergy 12:207-221, 1958

20. Pediatrics 27:790-799, 1961

21. Pediatric Clinics of North America 1:1019, 1954

22. Archives of Internal Medicine 115:155, 1965

23. Speer, Frederic, M. Allergy of the Nervous System. Springfield: C. C. Thomas, 1970

24. Speer, Frederic, MD Food Allergy. Second Edition, Boston: John Wright, 1983

25. British Medical Journal 282:2027-2029, June 20, 1981

26. American Journal of Nursing 80:262-265, February, 1980

27. Dr. James Braly, The Palm Beach Post, November 30, 1983

28. Annals of Allergy 51:574-580, December, 1983

29. Postgraduate Medicine 72(5)233-239, November, 1982

30. New England Journal of Medicine 307:895, 1982

31. Bahna, Sami L. DM and Douglas C. Heiner, MD. Allergies to Milk. New York: Grune and Stratten, 1980

32. American Family Practice 13(2)106-12, February, 1976

33. MCN: Maternal and Child Nursing 8:423-428, November-Decenber 1983

34. Speer, Frederic. MD Handbook of Clinical Allergy. Boston: John Wright, PSG, Inc. 1982

35. Consultant, June, 1980 p. 55-64

36. Journal of Family Practice 9(2)223-232, 1979

37. Deweese, David D. MD and William H. Saunders. Textbook of Otolaryngology, C. V. Mosby Co. 1964, p. 254-255

38. Lessof, M.H. Clinical Reactions to Food. New York: Wiley, 1983

39. Deweese. Op. cit. p. 81

40. John W. Gerrard, DM Food Allergy: New Perspectives. Springfield: Ill. C. C. Thomas, 1982

41. Annals of Allergy 42(2)69-72, February, 1979

42. Rowe, Albert H. MD Food Allergy: Its Manifestations, Diagnosis and Treatment. Philadelphia: Lea and Febinger, 1931, p. 354

43. Clin Rev Allergy 2:143-149, 1984

44. Journal of the American Medical Association 248(20)2627, November 26, 1982

45. The Lancet 2:437, 1980

46. American Family Physician 16(1)78, July, 1977

47. Quarterly Review of Allergy 6:157, 1952

48. American Journal of Psychiatry 130:6, June, 1973

49. Delaware Medical Journal 45:303-4, October, 1973

50. Adv. Biochem Psychopharmacol 22:535-48, 1980

51. Biological Psychiatry 16(12)3-19, December, 1981

52. Annals of Allergy 24:248-9, May, 1966

53. Speer, Frederic MD. Allergy of The Nervous System. Springfield, Ill: C.C. Thomas 1970

54. American Family Physician 11(2)88-94, February, 1975

55. Mackarness, Richard. Eating Dangerously: The Hazards of Allergies. New York: Harcourt, Brace, Jovanovich, 1976

56. Medical Tribune. Questions Patients Most Often Ask Their Doctors. New York: Bantam Books, 1983. p. 7-8

57. Annals of Allergy 47:124 August, 1981, Abstract 28

58. Rowe. Op. cit.

59. Faelten, Sharon. The Allergy Self-help Book. Emmaus, PA: Rodale Press, 1983

60. Annals of Allergy 48:166, March 1982

61. Journal of Clinical Psychiatry, 39(9)732 September, 1978

62. Philpott, William H. et al. Brain Allergies: The Psycho-Nutrient Connection. New Canaan, CT: Keats Publishing Co., 1980

63. Reed, Barbara PhD Food, Teens and Behavior. Manitowic, WI: Natural Press, 1983

64. Medical Times 96:759-73, August, 1968

65. Tuft, Louis MD and Harry Louis Mueller, MD Allergy in Children. Philadelphia: W. B. Saunders Co.

66. Acta Paediatrica Scandinavica 56:49-56, January, 1967

67. Annals of Allergy 26:33, 1968

68. Acta Paediatrica Scandinavica 54:101-115, March, 1965

69. The Lancet 1:339 February 12, 1977

70. Golos, Natalie and Frances Golos Golbitz. Coping With Your Allergies. New York: Simon and Schuster, 1979

71. Ludeman, Kate, PhD and Louise Henderson. Do-It-Yourself Allergy Analysis Handbook. New Canaan, CT: Keats Publishing Co., 1979

72. Journal of the International Academy of Preventive Medicine 7(3)32, November, 1982

INDEX